On-Call

X-Rays

MADE EASY

For Matilda, Evan, and our families
Iain and Amy

For my wife Judith, my parents, and my many radiology teachers
Nigel

Senior Commissioning Editor: Laurence Hunter
Development Editor: Carole McMurray
Project Manager: Kerrie-Ann McKinlay/Nancy Arnott
Designer: Charles Gray
Illustration Manager: Gillian Richards

On-Call

X-Rays

MADE EASY

Iain Au-Yong MA BMBCH MRCS FRCR

Consultant Radiologist, Kings Mill Hospital, Mansfield, UK; Formerly Specialist
Registrar, Queens Medical Centre, Nottingham, UK

Amy Au-Yong BSc (Hons) MB ChB

Foundation Doctor, Queens Medical Centre, Nottingham, UK

Nigel Broderick BS MB FRCP

Consultant Paediatric Radiologist, Nottingham University Hospitals; Training
Programme Director for East Midlands Deanery North (formerly Nottingham)
Radiology Training Scheme, Nottingham, England, UK

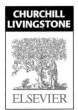

CHURCHILL
LIVINGSTONE

ELSEVIER

Edinburgh   London   New York   Oxford   Philadelphia   St Louis   Sydney   Toronto 2010

CHURCHILL
LIVINGSTONE
ELSEVIER

Main Edition ISBN 978-0-7020-3445-9

International ISBN 978-0-7020-3444-2

British Library Cataloguing in Publication Data
A catalogue record for this book is available from the British Library

Library of Congress Cataloging in Publication Data
A catalog record for this book is available from the Library of Congress

ELSEVIER your source for books, journals and multimedia in the health sciences
www.elsevierhealth.com

Working together to grow
libraries in developing countries
www.elsevier.com | www.bookaid.org | www.sabre.org

ELSEVIER   BOOK AID International   Sabre Foundation

The Publisher's policy is to use paper manufactured from sustainable forests

Printed in China

Contents

Introduction

Lines and Tubes

Chest X-Rays

Contents

Abdominal X-Rays

Bone X-Rays

Other

Paediatric X-Rays

About the authors

Iain Au-Yong is a newly appointed consultant in Radiology, who has passed the MRCS and FRCR exams. His clinical and radiological training has been wide-ranging and he has clinical experience in most of the major clinical specialties. This is his second book – he has written a popular MRCS revision text, which has sold many copies worldwide to surgical trainees. He has also contributed radiological and clinical material to other textbooks. He has extensive experience in lecturing and teaching medical students and junior doctors in a wide range of specialties. He has published several papers in prestigious peer-reviewed journals. He has also presented original research at international and national learned societies.

Amy Au-Yong is a foundation doctor who has retrained after initially working as a radiographer. She recognized the need for a book on interpretation of x-rays relevant to the on-call junior doctor, so came up with the original idea for this text. This book is aimed primarily at doctors at her stage of training and she has contributed useful clinical input to the book and ensured its content is appropriate for its audience. She has published papers in prestigious peer-reviewed journals and presented at international conferences.

Nigel Broderick is a Consultant Paediatric Radiologist to Nottingham University Hospitals, and Training Programme Director for the East Midlands Deanery North (formerly Nottingham) Radiology Training Scheme. He has extensive experience in the teaching of specialist registrars in radiology, junior doctors in a wide range of clinical specialties, and those in professions allied to medicine. With over twenty years' experience as a consultant, he is acutely aware how little he knew about interpreting plain films as a houseman and medical SHO, and how this skill is being persistently eroded by increasing reliance on cross-sectional imaging. He has published numerous papers in peer reviewed journals, presented original research at national and international meetings, and has been an invited speaker at events and courses organized by the Royal College of Radiologists and the Royal College of Surgeons.

Preface

Plain x-rays are often the first investigation carried out on patients presenting acutely, in all specialties. Their interpretation is of paramount importance, as accurate diagnosis will guide further investigation and management in these patients. Often, it will be the responsibility of a junior member of the medical team to request and interpret such investigations and timely involvement of senior, specialty and radiological colleagues may be necessary.

At the time of writing, in many countries, junior doctors' hours are being reduced as a legal requirement. With the same workforce, this necessitates an increase in work intensity, with resulting cross-cover of specialties in which basic radiographic appearances may not be familiar to the interpreting doctor. Prioritizing patient care is becoming increasingly important in the emergency setting.

Senior staff are also busier, and, particularly out of hours, obtaining their help to interpret every plain x-ray may be difficult. Disturbing your senior or a specialist in the middle of the night can be a daunting prospect and this book will aid identification of patients who require their immediate attention. It will also increase confidence in making such referrals, for which a succinct description of the radiograph concerned may be required.

This book provides a handy, portable aid to interpretation of a range of plain radiographs, many of which will have to be interpreted by the admitting or on-call ward doctor. The emphasis is on emergency plain x-ray appearances for which immediate management and senior help are necessary. The book will also help to guide initial further management, as well as guide the need for further imaging. We have not included any complex imaging so as not to confuse the reader and to impart a clear message, although the indications for requesting complex imaging, and answers to the radiologist's questions are covered.

The book's layout enables easy and quick reference, with a radiograph of each condition and a succinct description of the clinical signs, radiological signs and suggested further management of each life-threatening condition.

This book is aimed at junior doctors working in all specialties. Its use will also aid efficient and accurate referral across specialties. As emergency x-ray presentations are a common topic, and indeed pass–fail material for medical student finals, this book will also appeal to all clinical medical students. Its content may also be of interest to more senior doctors, and any health professional for whom interpretation of plain films in the acute setting is important, such as reporting radiographers and emergency nurse practitioners. It may also be helpful for radiology trainees as an introduction to 'hot reporting' films.

Acknowledgements

We would like to thank Laurence Hunter, Carole McMurray and Nancy Amott at Elsevier for their help and direction. Without their vision and support this project would not have been possible.

The authors would like to thank Kevin Hines for helping to locate radiographs and Craig Jobling, Maruti Kumaran, Gill Markham, Emma Lawrence and Godfrey Chatora for providing radiographs.

We would like to thank Rebecca Underwood for her organizational help.

Many thanks to Ijeoma Okonkwo for her help with reviewing the manuscript.

Many thanks to Medical Illustrations at King's Mill Hospital and Queen's Medical Centre for their assistance with the images.

Abbreviations and acronyms

AAA	Abdominal aortic aneurysm
A&E	Accident and Emergency
AXR	Abdominal x-ray
BP	Blood pressure
CML	Classic metaphyseal lesion
COPD	Chronic obstructive pulmonary disease
CR	Computed radiography
CRP	C-reactive protein
CT	Computed tomography
CTPA	CT pulmonary angiography
CVP	Central venous pressure
CXR	Chest x-ray
DR	Digital radiography
ECG	Electrocardiogram
ED	Emergency department
ERCP	Endoscopic retrograde cholangiopancreatography
ESR	Erythrocyte sedimentation rate
ET	Endotracheal
FBC	Full blood count
GI	Gastrointestinal
HDU	High dependency unit
IJV	Internal jugular vein
ITU	Intensive therapy unit
IVC	Inferior vena cava
IVU	Intravenous urogram
JVP	Jugular venous pressure
KUB	Kidneys, ureters and bladder
LBO	Large bowel obstruction
LMP	Last menstrual period
MDT	Multidisciplinary team meeting
MRCP	Magnetic resonance cholangiopancreatography
MRI	Magnetic resonance imaging
NAI	Non-accidental injury
NOF	Neck of femur
NG	Nasogastric
PC	Pelvicalyceal
PE	Pulmonary embolism
PUJ	Pelviureteric junction
SBO	Small bowel obstruction
SPN	Solitary pulmonary nodule
SpR	Specialist registrar
SCFE	Slipped capital femoral epiphysis
SUFE	Slipped upper femoral epiphysis

Abbreviations and acronyms

SVC	Superior vena cava
TB	Tuberculosis
US	Ultrasound
U+E	Urea and electrolytes
V/Q	Ventilation/perfusion (scan)
VUJ	Vesicoureteric junction
WCC	White cell count

Using this book

This book is designed to enable the reader to quickly recognize the appearances of life-threatening conditions. It is a comprehensive collection of conditions and radiographic appearances, which should be recognized by an on-call junior doctor.

It is, however, a guide, and there is no substitute for experience, so do involve your senior or radiology colleague if you are not sure. The appearances of pathologies can vary considerably between cases.

The layout is designed for easy reference. A large radiograph showing a classic appearance of the condition is presented at the beginning of each section accompanied by a line diagram based on this large radiograph outlining the pathology. Annotated close-ups of the radiological signs and appearances follow, and the area of interest in each close-up is demonstrated on the line diagram. The book is also cross-referenced to allow easy comparison with similar conditions.

We also provide tips for immediate management and when you need your senior to help you/when to refer and what to say, particularly about the radiology when referring, but these accounts are not comprehensive and are generally available in dedicated textbooks.

Introduction

How the radiograph is taken – basic CXR physics

The patient is placed adjacent to a cassette. Traditionally this contained a photographic film. Modern systems use computed radiography (CR) or digital radiography (DR) which can efficiently detect and capture the energy of x-rays to produce an image.

The x-ray source is 'aimed' at the patient and the x-rays travel in straight lines through the patient and darken the photographic film.

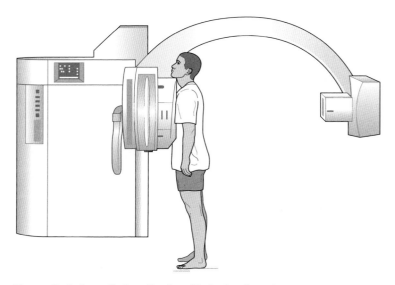

Diagram illustrating patient position for a PA chest radiograph.

Different tissues absorb varying amounts of x-rays as they pass through the patient; denser tissues absorb more x-rays than less dense ones.

The darkness of a tissue on the resulting radiograph is determined by how many x-rays have been absorbed as the beam passes through the patient. For example, bone absorbs most of the x-rays, so few make it through to darken the film and the bone appears white. On the other hand, the lungs, being composed mostly of air, absorb very few and the film is considerably darkened, the lungs thus appearing black on a radiograph.

Tissue densities

Different tissue densities have their own unique 'shades' on an x-ray:

- metal – bright white (arrow 1), in this case a pacemaker box
- bone – white (arrow 2)
- all soft tissues and fluid – grey (arrow 3)
- fat – grey/black (none seen on a CXR)
- air – black (arrow 4).

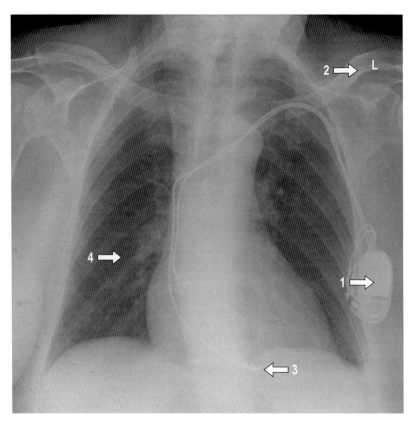

Chest radiograph of patient with permanent pacemaker illustrating different densities.

Organs can be seen if they are of a different density or thickness than those adjacent to them. For example, the outline of the heart is well seen on a CXR because the heart is of soft tissue/water density and adjacent to the lungs (air density).

Organs of the same density but different thickness can be seen next to each other but this is more difficult – this is why individual organs are more difficult to see on AXRs (see Chapter 28).

Silhouette signs

When areas of different density are adjacent to one another they produce an edge on the radiograph (e.g. the hemidiaphragm next to the lung base). The best way to understand this phenomenon is to explain it using the CXR as an example.

On a normal CXR the right heart border 'edge' is clearly seen. This is because it is of soft tissue density and is adjacent to the air density of the lung. The same principle applies with the hemidiaphragm (also soft tissue density), which is adjacent to the lung bases (air dense) and therefore the well-defined 'edge' of the hemidiaphragm can easily be seen.

In pathological processes these edges can be lost, enabling exact anatomical localization of the abnormality. This principle is called the silhouette sign.

A good example of this is right middle lobe pneumonia. The soft tissue/water density heart border 'edge' is no longer seen as it is now adjacent to the water density pneumonia in the lung. As there is no difference in density between the two areas they now appear to merge into one. The disappearance of this edge combined with the knowledge that the right middle lobe lies adjacent to the right heart border confirms that the pathology is in the middle lobe.

Another example is the loss of the hemidiaphragm 'edge' on a CXR of a patient with a pleural effusion. The soft tissue/water density of the hemidiaphragm is now adjacent to the water density of the effusion and the clear outline of the hemidiaphragm is lost.

This same principle can be used to explain a useful diagnostic feature of pneumonias on the CXR – the air bronchogram. Normally, a bronchus is not seen within the lung as it contains air and is adjacent to the alveoli, which also contain air. If that section of the lung develops pneumonia, the air-containing bronchus within the pneumonia is now adjacent to alveoli that contain fluid and can therefore now be seen as a branching structure – an air bronchogram.

Also note that pulmonary vessels are clearly seen against normal lung (water against air) – this is what is seen in the normal hilum – but they disappear in a segment of pneumonia (water against water).

See pneumonia (Chapter 8) and collapse (Chapter 17) sections for applications of this phenomenon.

Requesting radiological investigations – a guide

This is a quick guide to the things you need to know when requesting radiology. Please read this section as it may help you avoid misunderstandings with radiology when on call!

Radiation doses

It is useful to know the radiation dose of common plain film examinations for a few reasons. Patients may ask, and it is also undesirable to request unnecessary high-dose examinations on young patients, particularly if the gonadal dose is high. The radiographer performing the investigation may challenge the indication, particularly in high-dose investigations on young patients if it is not clear from the request card why it is indicated, so make this clear when requesting.

The Royal College of Radiologists publication 'Making the best use of clinical radiology services' [1] is a good guide as to which clinical indications are appropriate for each radiological investigation.

One CXR is equivalent in dose to 3 days of background radiation in Cornwall. The dose is low as the chest contains a lot of air (lungs) so less radiation is absorbed.

Other doses in numbers of CXRs (approximate) are as follows: [2]
- cervical spine – 1.5
- pelvis – 14
- abdomen – 16
- thoracic spine – 24
- lumbar spine – 60.

As you can see, all plain films are not equal in dose. An AXR is much higher than a CXR. Lumbar spine radiographs, which are requested very commonly for patients with suspected intervertebral disc pathology where the diagnostic yield is almost negligible, are associated with a significant radiation dose.

Complex examinations such as a barium enema carry a dose equivalent to 120 or so CXRs, and CT is also as high as this so the radiation dose becomes even more relevant.

The importance of this is that the theoretical risk of fatal cancer increases with radiation dose. One study estimated the risk with whole-body CT to be 0.08% [3].

Filling out the request card

The following need to be completed in full on a request card. Otherwise your request may be rejected.

Patient details including date of birth and a second identifier such as address/hospital number are required in order to check the patient's identity in the radiology department and also to record the examination on the Radiology Information System. Remember the patient may be confused.

A pertinent **clinical history** and **relevant past and ongoing medical history** will also be needed. This is a *legal requirement* before the radiographer is allowed to x-ray the patient. So don't get upset if the radiographer bleeps you when you are busy to reject your request because the details are not filled out comprehensively or legibly. Also, remember that although you will probably be the first to see this radiograph, you are simultaneously making a referral to a radiologist for their opinion (report). Their report will be more meaningful if you have provided a clinical context for the findings on the plain film. For example, if you know the patient has cancer this is always relevant.

If the patient is female and of childbearing age add the pregnancy status. It is not a good idea to unknowingly irradiate an unborn fetus as the radiation has teratogenic effects. In pregnant patients undergoing necessary investigations dose reduction measures may need to be taken and a radiologist is often involved in decision-making. The pregnancy test is also a useful diagnostic test in patients of childbearing age presenting with low abdominal pain and should always be remembered in their diagnostic work-up.

This may be a good place to explain the 28-day and 10-day rules. The 28-day rule is applied to high-dose examinations which also irradiate the uterus. The investigation should take place within 28 days of the patient's last period. Therefore asking the patient about the last menstrual period (LMP) is important in this assessment. The 10-day rule does not really apply to plain films but may apply to your subsequent request for high-dose complex imaging. If the test is very high dose to the uterus the patient should have the test within 10 days of the last period (as the patient is more likely to conceive after ovulation, in the second half of the cycle).

Put your name and bleep number on the card legibly so the radiographer or radiologist can contact you if they identify a problem that needs urgent attention (most of the conditions in this book!). Sign the request (legal requirement). Knowing the responsible consultant is helpful.

How can the patient travel? Do you need a portable film? It's amazing how much trouble this can cause if the porter comes up to your ward with a chair and bed transport is required – result: delay in your patient's test.

Call the radiographer in advance if the test is particularly urgent or needs to be done portably.

The patient journey

Once you have requested the plain film, the patient will be put on a list to come down to the department for their test. If the test is urgent it can be arranged more quickly.

The patient will come to the department or have their radiograph done portably. Most hospitals now have picture archiving communications systems (PACS). Images are stored electronically for review on workstations and PC monitors. The radiograph will also be put on a 'hot reporting' system for the duty radiologist to report. The hot reporting room will have a radiologist in it during the day so if you are concerned about a certain plain film appearance then the hot reporting radiologist is a good source of advice on interpretation and appropriate further investigation. On-call radiology is becoming busier and often there is an on-call radiologist in the hospital out of hours to help you, but enlist your own senior first as they may also be better placed to assess the radiograph in the context of the patient.

References

[1] Making the best use of clinical radiology services. 6th ed. Ref No: BFCR(07)10. Royal College of Radiologists; 2007.
[2] Warren-Forward HM, Haddaway MJ, Temperton DH, McCall IW. Dose area product readings for fluoroscopic and plain film examinations, including an analysis of the source of variation for barium enema examinations. BJR 1998;71:961–7.
[3] Brenner DJ, Elliston CD. Estimated radiation risks potentially associated with full-body CT screening. Radiology 2004;232:735–8.

Preparing patients for CT

This section has been included as this is very often the next test to be organized if you spot one of the abnormalities described in this book.

Having the correct information to hand and proper patient preparation will help to ensure that there are no unnecessary delays with scanning your patient.

Contrast media

Intravenous contrast

Most patients will require intravenous contrast. This gives a lot of useful information about the vascularity of organs and of pathologies and is necessary to enable your radiological colleague to make a diagnosis for you. In order to be able to administer contrast, the following need to be determined:

- Is the patient allergic to iodinated contrast media?
- Is the patient a diabetic on metformin? (If so discuss with a radiologist.)
- Does the patient have renal impairment? This means having the patient's most recent U+E to hand before picking up the phone to call the radiologist. Intravenous contrast in renal impairment can cause contrast-induced nephropathy.

If the patient does have renal impairment the risk of contrast administration needs to be balanced against the extra information available from administration of contrast and this needs to be a shared decision between a senior clinical doctor and the duty radiologist.

Oral contrast

Patients for abdominal CT also require oral contrast. This is a radio-opaque medium which opacifies the lumen of the bowel to aid interpretation. A time interval is left between ingestion and scanning to enable it to traverse as much of the bowel as possible. Also if a perforation is suspected, passage of contrast into the peritoneal cavity clinches the diagnosis (although this is uncommon).

Oral contrast can be drunk by the patient or put down a nasogastric tube. If a patient is strictly nil by mouth (e.g. bowel obstruction or immediately postoperative) it may cause vomiting. If the patient is preoperative (e.g. presenting with an acute abdomen and being starved in case they need an operation) the anaesthetist may not consider oral contrast to be contraindicated but you should check with your senior/anaesthetic colleague if you are unsure.

Other preparation and information

The patient requires intravenous access for intravenous contrast. A green 18G cannula is required for angiographic CT such as CT pulmonary angiography (CTPA).

The location of the patient and mode of transport should be made known to staff at the CT unit, so that appropriate portering services can be arranged.

A medical escort should be provided if the patient is unstable. The porter does not want to be dealing with a cardiac arrest.

In young females of childbearing age (11–50) pregnancy status is very important as CT examinations are high dose. The date of the patient's last menstrual period should be recorded on the request card.

If any intervention is going to be needed, a clotting screen and FBC results are also required.

The plain film findings may need to be discussed, particularly when imaging for suspected pulmonary embolism (see Chapter 24).

System for presenting plain films in exams or on ward rounds

This is a brief guide on presentation of any plain film.

- Presentation should start with **what type of film is being described** and patient's **name**, **age**, and **sex**.

'This is a PA chest radiograph on Frederick Bloggs, a 56-year-old man.'

- If appropriate, comment on whether the film is of good **technical quality** (see Chapter 6)

'The film is not rotated, is well inspired and of good penetration.'

- **Describe any abnormality** which initially catches your eye, much as you would describe signs and symptoms in a patient you had just assessed clinically and were presenting.

'There is a rounded, well-defined, approximately 3 cm solitary mass in the apex of the right lung.'

- If you don't see anything, **check the review areas** for that type of film (see Chapters 7 and 28), and if an abnormality becomes apparent, start to describe it.
- Describe **relevant negatives**, or other **relevant positive findings** on the film. You may wish to look at relevant review areas at this stage.

'No evidence of rib destruction.'

- Summarize and give a main diagnosis with or without a differential diagnosis.

'Overall appearances are in keeping with a bronchogenic carcinoma in the right upper lobe. Differentials include causes of a solitary pulmonary nodule, including a lung metastasis, particularly if the patient has a known primary tumour.'

- Briefly outline **further management**. This will usually include reviewing previous films if available, resuscitative measures if appropriate, further imaging and referral to a specialist team if appropriate.

'I would review previous films to see if the lesion is new or enlarging; referral to the lung cancer multidisciplinary team meeting with a view to cross-sectional imaging is recommended.'

Lines and tubes

1 Nasogastric tubes

Background

Nasogastric (NG) tubes are placed for a number of medical reasons. These include decompression of the gastrointestinal tract in a patient with intestinal obstruction and for feeding in patients who cannot safely swallow. Traditional methods for confirmation of the position of the tube such as insufflation of gas and pH measurements have been shown to be unreliable, and the gold standard for determining the position of the tip of an NG tube is a CXR.

The stakes are high, particularly if the tube has been inserted for the purpose of feeding. If the NG tube does not enter the oesophagus and progress to the stomach, the likely alternative route and destination is the bronchial tree and lung, usually via the more steeply inclined right main bronchus. Introducing a high volume of feed into the lung via such a malpositioned tube can cause pneumonia, and death of patients following this error has occurred.

The responsibility for ensuring the position of the tube is correct before feeding often falls upon the on-call junior doctor, who may be asked by a nursing colleague to confirm correct placement.

Remember, if you are not sure your senior or radiology colleague is there to help you.

Lines and tubes

Radiological features

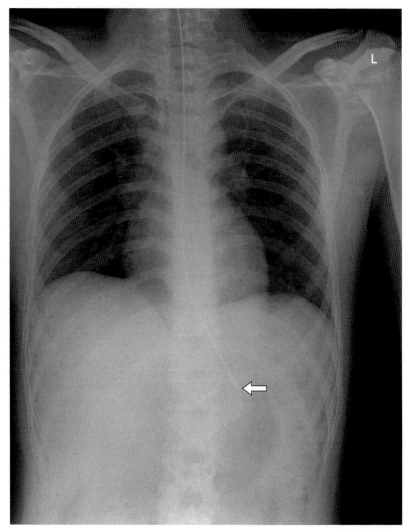

Fig. 1.1 This patient has an appropriately positioned NG tube. This is a simple exercise in anatomy.

An NG tube will go down either the oesophagus or trachea. Remember the anatomy of the oesophagus. It is a midline posterior mediastinal structure, which enters the abdominal cavity at the level of the T10 vertebra. So for the tube to be correctly placed within the stomach its tip must be below the diaphragm. Any tube whose tip is above the diaphragm is inappropriately placed.

This tube terminates in the region of the stomach (arrow).

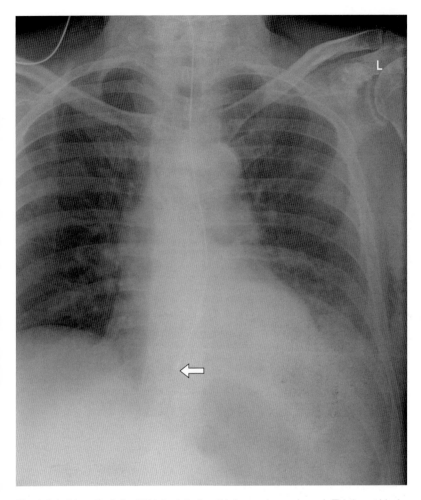

Fig. 1.2 In this patient, the NG tube is in the distal oesophagus (arrow). This is not ideal as the patient is at an increased risk of aspiration. This tube needs repositioning.

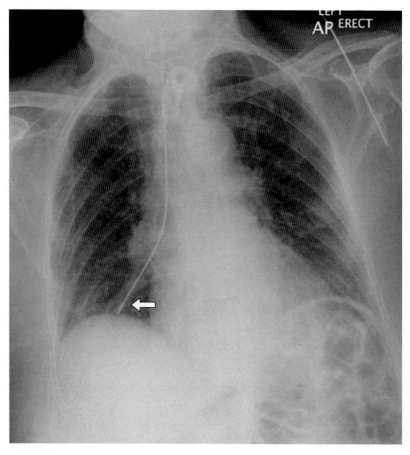

Fig. 1.3 This patient has an NG tube in the lung (arrow). The tip of the NG tube is projected over the lung having travelled via the right main bronchus to get there. Remember: if it's above the diaphragm it's in the wrong place.

Remember that the only completely reliable method of ensuring the NG tube is positioned correctly is a CXR. This is more accurate than pH measurement or gas insufflation.

Further reading

Kunis K. Confirmation of nasogastric tube placement. Am J Crit Care 2007;16(1):19.

2 Endotracheal tubes

Background

Endotracheal (ET) tubes are placed within the trachea as a definitive airway to allow mechanical ventilation in a patient who cannot maintain their own airway due to, for example, a low level of consciousness, in a cardiac arrest situation or during anaesthesia. Patients in intensive care units are frequently intubated and ventilated.

The CXR is the gold standard for determining placement of the tube. A knowledge of anatomy is the key for interpretation.

Radiological features

There are only two directions in which the ET tube can go: the trachea, or oesophagus. The latter is of course undesirable but very difficult to diagnose on a frontal CXR as the oesophagus lies immediately posterior to the trachea within the mediastinum and the CXR is a 2D representation of the thorax. Excessive air in the upper GI tract can be a sign of accidental intubation of the oesophagus.

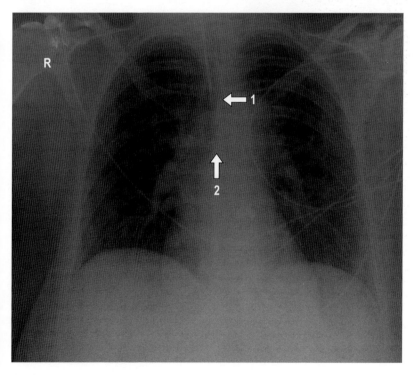

Fig. 2.1 This patient has an appropriately positioned ET tube (arrow 1). The ET tube tip should be approximately 5 cm, or a few vertebral body heights above the carina (arrow 2).

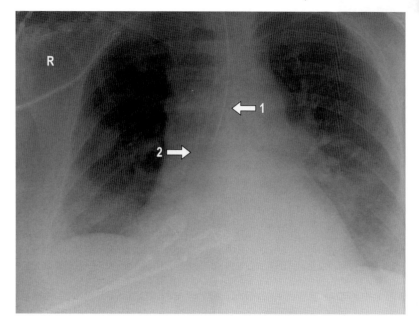

Fig. 2.2 When checking the position of the ET tube, always check for accidental intubation of the right main bronchus. Identification of the carina (tracheal bifurcation) is again key for interpretation (arrow 1). Anatomically, the right main bronchus is steeper than the left, so an ET tube that has been inserted too far will preferentially enter the right main bronchus (this is also the reason that inhaled foreign bodies preferentially enter the right main bronchus).

In this patient the tube is clearly distal to the carina in the right main bronchus (arrow 2).

If the tube is left in this position, the left lung will collapse (and turn white; see Chapter 9). This case illustrates why looking at the tubes and lines first is sensible as often they are the cause of a lung abnormality.

3 Central lines

Background

Central lines or central venous pressure (CVP) lines are placed to allow access to the central venous circulation. They have several functions, such as venous access for administration of drugs/fluids/feeding and monitoring. Several other types of intravenous catheter exist and principles for interpretation of radiographs following insertion of these lines are the same. Examples include Permcaths in dialysis patients, Hickman lines for patients who require long-term antibiotics and portacaths for patients who inject antibiotics or other medications long term.

They are placed in a wide range of patients, in ITU and the ward setting in both medical and surgical patients.

Radiological features

There are two main objectives when interpreting radiographs following placement of a CVP line:
1. Is line placement and position correct?
2. Are there any complications? The commonest are pneumothorax and mediastinal haematoma secondary to vessel damage.

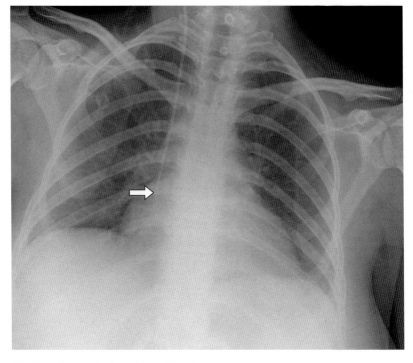

Fig. 3.1A Appropriately positioned CVP line.

The two routes of access are the internal jugular vein in the neck (jugular CVP line) or the subclavian vein below the clavicle.

This patient has an internal jugular central line. In this case, the line traverses the internal jugular vein, the right brachiocephalic vein, then the superior vena cava, which forms the right hand border of the upper mediastinum. The appropriate point for the tip of the line is the superior vena cava (SVC) or right atrium (upper right heart) (arrow).

More rarely, a left-sided central line may pass into the left side of the mediastinum indicating a left-sided SVC. Normally a left internal jugular line would enter the left brachiocephalic vein, then the SVC on the right (see Fig. 3.1b).

A subclavian line would end in the same place but starts in the upper lateral chest and traverses the brachiocephalic vein before entering the SVC.

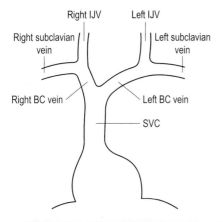

Fig. 3.1B Line diagram indicating relevant venous anatomy for interpretation. SVC = superior vena cava, IJV = internal jugular vein, BC = brachiocephalic.

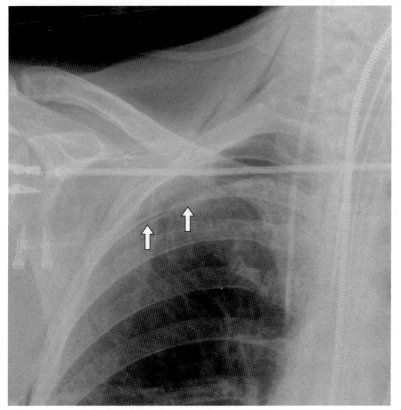

Fig. 3.2 Pneumothorax complicating right internal jugular CVP line insertion. In this different patient there is a subtle apical pneumothorax following the contour of the posterior third rib (arrows). The risk of pneumothorax is higher with subclavian central lines compared with the jugular route of insertion. See Chapter 18 for more on pneumothorax interpretation.

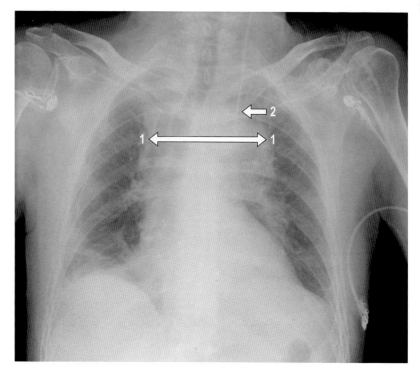

Fig. 3.3 Widened mediastinum following CVP line insertion. The presence of a wide mediastinum raises concern about mediastinal haematoma (arrow 1). However, AP films, supine AP films and rotated films can cause magnification of the mediastinum and should be interpreted with caution. Note the left internal jugular central line (arrow 2). See Chapter 23 for more on the widened mediastinum.

If this appearance is seen, ensure the patient is stable, and promptly discuss the case with your senior. Cross-sectional imaging may be required to make the diagnosis.

4 Permanent pacemakers

Background

Cardiac pacing is an established and effective treatment for cardiac arrhythmias and placement of a permanent pacemaker is a common procedure in hospitals. It may be one of your tasks as a junior doctor to arrange check x-rays for such patients and interpret them.

Complications following placement of a permanent pacemaker device are relatively common, 20% in one study [1], and their detection is improved by a knowledge of the commonest things that can go wrong.

Pneumothorax and lead malposition are the commonest complications and they are illustrated below.

Correct placement

The commonest pacing systems are dual-chamber and single-chamber pacing devices.

A good understanding of cardiac anatomy is helpful for interpretation (see Chapter 7).

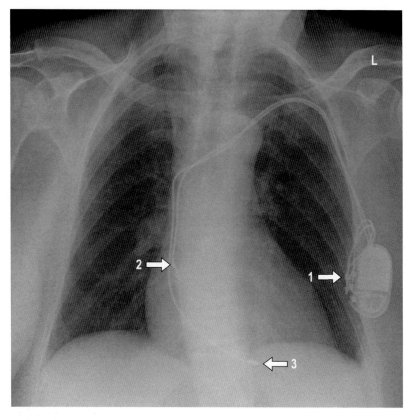

Fig. 4.1 Correctly positioned dual-chamber permanent pacemaker device. The pacemaker box is positioned subcutaneously, usually in the left upper thorax (arrow 1).

In a dual-chamber device there are two pacing leads whose tips should generally be in the right atrium (arrow 2) and right ventricle (arrow 3), respectively.

Interpretation is easy – with a dual-chamber pacing device look to see if the tips are in the right atrium and ventricle. If not they are likely to be malpositioned. Particularly look to see if the lead is outside the heart and great vessels (which suggests the lead has gone through cardiac or vessel wall to get there).

In a single-chamber device the single lead tip is in the right ventricle. Imagine this pacemaker without the atrial lead present. See Fig. 4.3 for an example of a single lead pacemaker.

Lead malposition

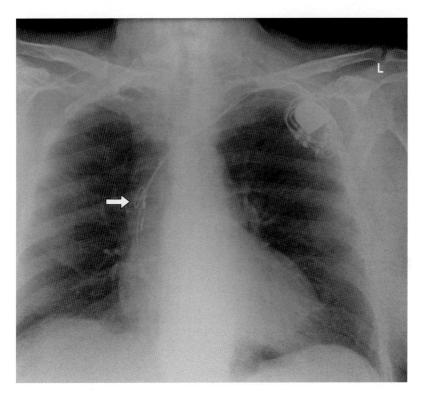

Fig. 4.2 Malpositioned pacemaker device. This patient's atrial lead is coiled in the superior vena cava. It requires repositioning (arrow).

Complications

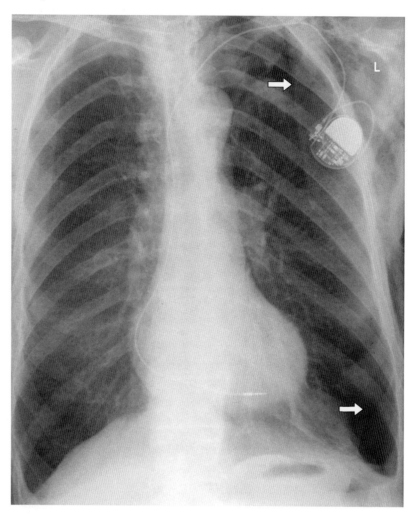

Fig. 4.3 Left pneumothorax and surgical emphysema complicating single-chamber pacemaker insertion. Pneumothorax is the commonest complication of pacemaker insertion (arrows). See Chapter 18 for a further account of the appearances.

Other things to look for

Look for discontinuity of the pacemaker leads, which might suggest a fracture of the lead. This tends to happen as a late complication but you may save the patient's life with a sharp eye. Many patients who present in the on-call (or outpatient) setting have had pacemakers placed several years ago which may now have developed a problem.

Reference

[1] Grier D, Cook PG, Hartnell GG. Chest radiographs after permanent pacing, are they really necessary? Clin Radiol 1990;42(4):244–9.

Further reading

For a more detailed account of the radiological appearances:
Burney K, Burchard F, Papouchado M, Wilde P. Cardiac pacing systems and implantable cardiac defibrillators (ICDs): a radiological perspective of equipment, anatomy and complications. Clin Radiol 2004;59:699–708.

5 Chest drains

Background

Chest drains are placed for the drainage of pleural space collections. These may include pneumothoraces (Chapter 18), pleural effusions (Chapter 20) and haemothoraces in trauma patients.

Chest drains may be either large-bore or fine-bore (pigtail drain), the latter being the type most often inserted in the radiology department under ultrasound guidance. Large-bore chest drains are inserted using a blind technique so the position should be carefully scrutinized on a CXR. Remember that ultrasound-guided drains can also be misplaced.

Radiological features

CXRs are performed for a number of reasons:
1. To ensure satisfactory placement.
2. To monitor the response of the pathology to drainage – serial CXRs are often performed in these patients. Often the duration of tube drainage is determined by the CXR appearances.
3. For detection of complications.

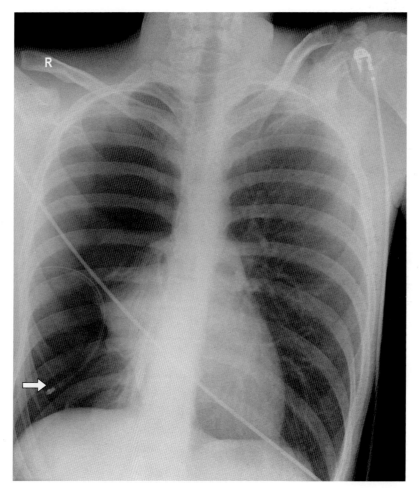

Fig. 5.1 This patient has an appropriately positioned drain within a large right pneumothorax (arrow).

The tip of a chest drain is often difficult to localize, because a frontal CXR depicts the chest in one plane only.

If the tip is projected over the heart, mediastinum or opposite hemithorax, this does not automatically mean it is malpositioned but this possibility should be considered.

Correlate the findings with clinical function of the drain, the patient's clinical indices and information relating to the procedure in the patient's notes/radiology system, and consider cross-sectional imaging if you need to be sure of the position.

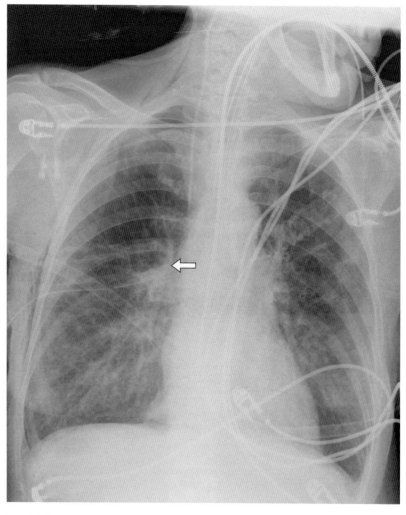

Fig. 5.2 The difficulty in localization is illustrated here – this patient actually had a chest drain in the lung (arrow) as demonstrated later on a CT scan. If the drain is projected over the lung, it may be correctly placed in the pleural space or in the lung.

One clue as to incorrect placement in the lung is the failure of a lung to reinflate over several days – caused by a bronchopleural fistula. In this circumstance CT has been shown to be more sensitive than a CXR alone [1] but remember that a CXR is simpler to perform and adequate in most cases. A lateral film may also help for further localization.

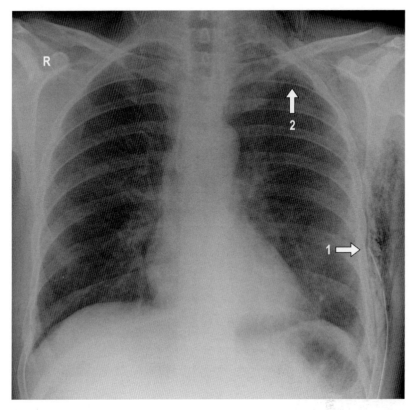

Fig. 5.3 This is the sort of circumstance in which a CXR is helpful: this drain is clearly not in far enough (arrow 1) and not in the pleural space – it is in the soft tissues of the chest. There is soft tissue surgical emphysema. Note the small left apical pneumothorax (arrow 2).

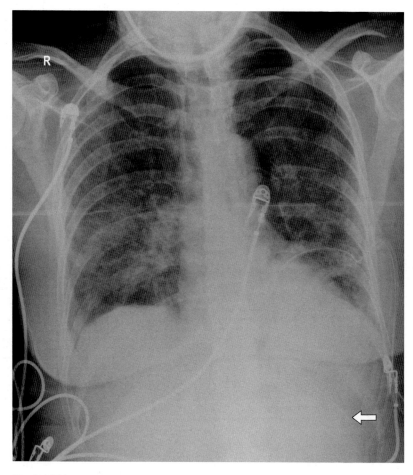

Fig. 5.4 This patient's chest drain tip has found its way into the abdomen (arrow). Follow the tube along its entire course. This is not as uncommon as you might imagine.

Reference

[1] Lim KE, Tai SC, Chan CY, et al. Diagnosis of malpositioned chest tubes after emergency tube thoracostomy – is computed tomography more accurate than chest radiograph? Clin Imaging 2005;29:401–5.

Chest x-rays

6

Technical factors in CXR interpretation

Technical factors are very important as they can mimic pathology. They may cause normal lung to appear white on the radiograph, mimicking other pathologies such as infection and heart failure.

This chapter provides a checklist of technical factors to be considered before interpreting the film, and an accompanying explanation of how they affect the resulting image.

Remember that in an unwell patient, a suboptimal film may be all that it is possible to obtain and important pathology may be overlooked if these films are dismissed.

Demographics

Check the patient's name, age and sex – this often changes the differential diagnosis. It is also important that you are interpreting the correct patient's film!

Projection: posteroanterior (PA) versus anteroposterior (AP)

See also page 3.

The ideal view is PA (left radiograph in Fig. 6.1) and is taken with the patient sitting or standing upright, with the front of their chest against the cassette. The x-rays go through the patient from their back through to the front, hence the description PA. For this view, the patient moves their scapulae laterally away from the chest wall by bringing their arms to each side of the x-ray machine. Performing this view requires the patient to be reasonably fit and well.

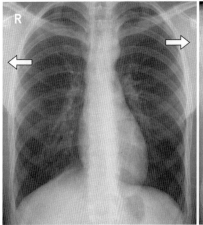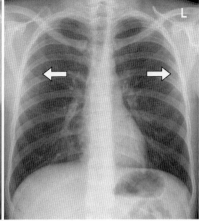

Fig. 6.1 PA (left) and AP (right) views.

The AP view (right radiograph in Fig. 6.1) is taken with the cassette behind the patient. This is the technique used in portable films and for patients who are not well enough to sit or stand upright, such as ill inpatients.

Because the heart and mediastinal structures are relatively anterior in the chest, their true size is best depicted on a PA film, where they are closer to the cassette. For this reason the heart size and mediastinal width are most accurately assessed on a PA film – they are magnified on an AP film.

To determine which projection you are assessing, first look to see if the radiographer has marked the film AP or PA. If the scapulae are overlapping the chest wall (arrows, Fig. 6.1 right) the film is AP. If they are not and are excluded, the film is PA (arrows, Fig. 6.1 left).

An important parameter to assess when looking at the CXR is the cardiothoracic ratio. This is the ratio of heart diameter at its widest point to thoracic diameter at its widest point. If this is over 0.5 on a PA film the heart is enlarged in its transverse diameter. This is a key assessment to make in heart failure (see Chapter 26). Heart size cannot always be reliably assessed on an AP film.

Erect versus supine

PA films are taken erect. Patients may be supine for AP/portable films.

It is important to remember that air rises and fluid settles dependently with patients in different positions. This can be used to diagnostic advantage, and should be remembered when interpreting films.

For assessment of pneumoperitoneum, an erect film needs to be taken as this will allow free gas in the abdomen to collect under the diaphragm. A patient with a suspected pneumoperitoneum should sit upright for at least 5 minutes before a film is taken for this indication (see Chapter 27).

Pleural space collections such as pneumothoraces and effusions also do not look the same on supine and erect films (see Chapters 18 and 20).

Adequacy

The whole chest should be included on the radiograph. This should include both costophrenic angles and lung apices, and the head should not be slumped over the mediastinum.

Side marker

Check the side marker: the heart cannot be assumed to be on the left as in patients with dextrocardia it is on the right.

Rotation

Rotation causes a problem as it makes one lung look whiter than the other and also can cause apparent widening of the mediastinum.

Rotation can be assessed by measuring the distance between each medial clavicle and the spinous process at this level. In a well-centred film these

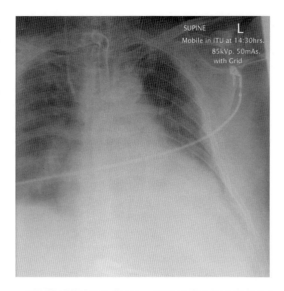

Fig. 6.2 This film is inadequate as much of the right hemithorax has not been included on it. Additionally it is blurred as the patient has moved.

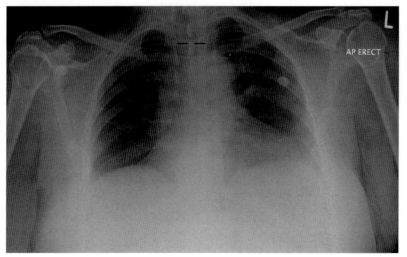

Fig. 6.3 Rotation.

distances should be equidistant. In a rotated film these distances are different (black lines in Fig. 6.3).

Penetration/Exposure

To create the picture, the x-ray source has to be 'switched on' at a certain power setting by the radiographer. If this is done for too short a time, the film is underexposed as not enough x-rays have penetrated the patient to darken the film and this can make the lungs look whiter than they actually are.

Conversely, with too much exposure the lungs will look too black and subtle pathology in them may be masked. Issues with penetration are less common now with the widespread use of CR/DR.

To determine adequate penetration look at the cervical spine and the thoracic spine behind the heart. If the penetration is right you will just about be able to see the vertebral bodies projected behind the heart, and you should see the intervertebral discs at the level of the upper cervical spine.

The rotated film above (Fig. 6.3) is also poorly penetrated. The vertebral bodies at the level of the heart cannot be seen.

Inspiration

The best film is taken when the patient has taken a good breath in. This fills the lungs with air. If the lungs are not inflated due to a poor inspiration, then they appear falsely white.

A well-inspired film is one in which six or more anterior ribs are seen above the hemidiaphragms bilaterally.

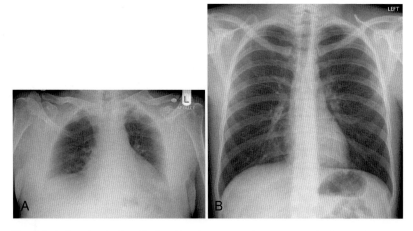

Fig. 6.4 A: Poor inspiration. **B:** Good inspiration. See the differences in the lung bases.

Lateral films

A film can be taken with the patient standing side-on to the beam for localization of lesions. Interpretation of lateral films is complex and is not covered in this text.

7 System for interpretation of the CXR

This chapter is a checklist of all the places to look on a CXR once you have checked the technical quality of the radiograph. A sound knowledge of anatomy is vital and key anatomical structures are highlighted.

Always look for old films of your patient for comparison. This will help you determine if an abnormality is an acute or chronic problem. CXR abnormalities which have been there for years are seldom of any importance. You will see examples of the importance of looking at old films in the ensuing chapters.

After checking the technical quality, ensure any lines and tubes are correctly positioned. Malposition of tubes or lines may be the cause of other abnormalities on the film. See the 'Lines and tubes' section for examples.

If any abnormality is obviously present, at this point, describe it fully.

Important areas for review are described in this chapter.

There are many mnemonics to remember what to check – just as long as you look at everything it does not matter which one you use, if any.

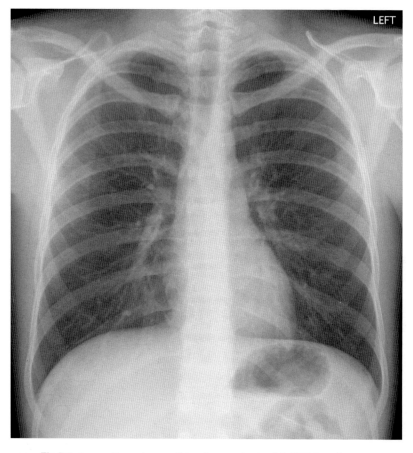

Fig 7.1 Areas of importance will be discussed using this CXR for reference.

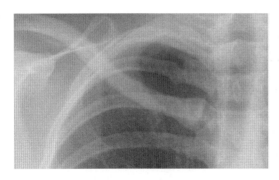

Fig. 7.2 Look at the lungs. In particular, look at the apices. There are a lot of overlapping bony structures here which can make interpretation difficult. Tumours are often missed here (see Chapter 15). Some pathologies have a predilection for the apices, such as TB (see Chapter 11).

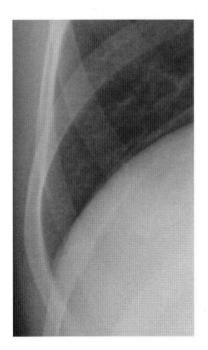

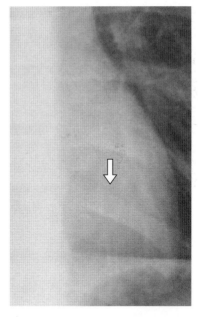

Fig. 7.3 The costophrenic angles are another important place to look. Many pathologies start here. Septal lines in early heart failure are found here (see Chapter 26), as are pleural effusions, which blunt the costophrenic angles (see Chapter 20).

Fig. 7.4 There is a considerable amount of lung (left lower lobe) hidden behind the heart. Cancers can be hidden here; look also for left lower lobe collapse (see Chapter 17) and consolidation (see Chapter 8). Loss of the contour of the hemidiaphragm behind the heart (arrow) can be a clue, so always look for this structure.

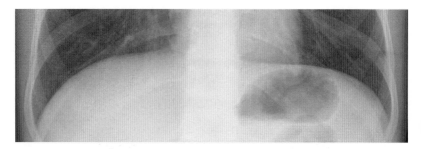

Fig. 7.5 Remember the hemidiaphragms. The right hemidiaphragm is normally higher than the left as it has the liver underneath it. Look for free air under the hemidiaphragms on an erect CXR (see Chapter 27). A grossly raised hemidiaphragm may be due to diaphragmatic paralysis caused by a phrenic nerve palsy. Subpulmonic effusions can cause an apparent raised hemidiaphragm (see Chapter 20). They generally occur in patients lying supine or semi-erect for long periods.

There is lung tissue in the posterior costophrenic region below the diaphragmatic outline on a PA film – another important review area.

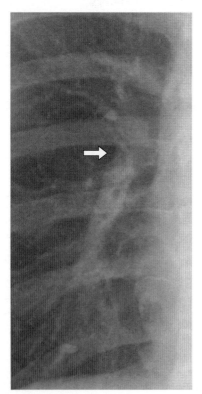

Fig. 7.6 Don't forget the pulmonary hila. These contain pulmonary vessels (arteries and veins) as well as lymph nodes and bronchi (arrow).

Abnormalities of any of these structures can lead to enlargement of the hilum, e.g. dilated pulmonary arteries in pulmonary hypertension, lung cancer affecting the bronchus and enlarged lymph nodes in malignancy or certain infections such as TB.

The lateral margin of the hila should be concave in outline. Bulging convexity of the hilar outline should be considered abnormal.

The left hilum is normally a little higher than the right. If the hila are in the wrong position it may indicate loss of volume in one lung.

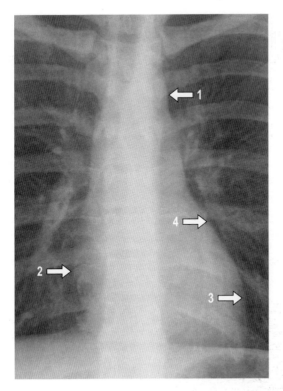

Fig. 7.7 The heart and mediastinum are important. Look at the transverse diameter of the heart, which should be half or less of the diameter of the bony thorax on a PA film. The mediastinum should not be widened. It should be less than 7 cm on a PA film. Widening raises the concern of aortic dissection (see Chapter 23), although again enlargement of any structure within the mediastinum may lead to widening. Look at the aortic knuckle (arrow 1), a posterior mediastinal structure. Loss of its contour may indicate posterior pathology, or a problem with the aorta itself.

Be familiar with the cardiac chambers. The right heart border is formed by the right atrium (arrow 2). The left heart border is formed by the left ventricle caudally (arrow 3) and the left atrium (arrow 4) more superiorly. Remember that the right ventricle is anterior and therefore its edge is not seen.

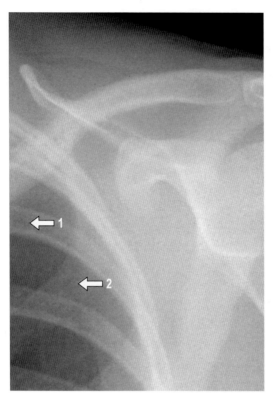

Fig. 7.8 Remember to look at the bones. Look at the ribs, clavicles and shoulders. Look for missing and fractured ribs.

Remember the difference between a posterior and anterior rib as this is important for description. Posterior ribs are horizontal (arrow 1) and anterior ribs are directed inferiorly (arrow 2).

Think of the bucket handle model of respiration you learned in physiology. In expiration the front of the rib slopes downwards and when you breathe in the ribs become more horizontal to increase the AP diameter of the chest.

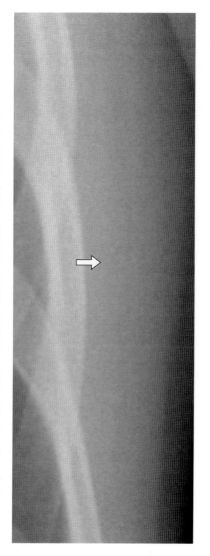

Fig. 7.9 Don't forget the soft tissues (arrow). These may contain air or may be swollen.

8 Pneumonia

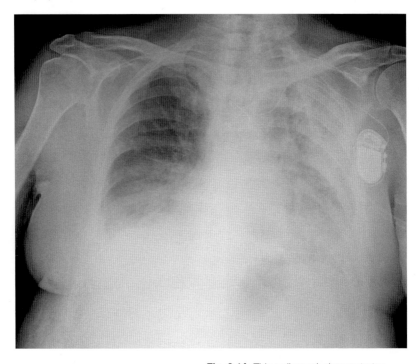

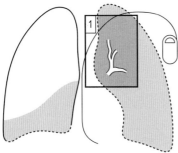

Fig. 8.1A This radiograph demonstrates bilateral pneumonia, worse on the left than on the right. Note the air bronchograms on the left. The patient also has a permanent pacemaker in situ.

Background

This is an extremely common presentation to the on-call doctor. It can present on admission wards as community-acquired pneumonia or complicate a ward stay in any patient – those undergoing surgery are at particular risk of postoperative infection, particularly with thoracoabdominal surgery as the cough reflex is impaired and respiration is often limited by pain.

Clinical features

Symptoms

The symptoms include shortness of breath (SOB), productive cough (green sputum), haemoptysis, fever, rigors and pleuritic chest pain.

Signs

There are signs of local consolidation (coarse crackles, bronchial breathing, increased vocal resonance).

Differential diagnosis

This condition has both a clinical and radiological differential diagnosis. The diagnosis is made with a combination of clinical and radiological findings.

Clinical differentials to consider

- Pulmonary embolus – pleuritic chest pain/SOB/haemoptysis but sudden onset, usually no fever. The CXR is usually normal (see Chapter 24), but see also below.
- Cardiac failure – SOB, sudden onset; often many specific signs and symptoms such as orthopnoea/paroxysmal nocturnal dyspnoea (PND), displaced apex, pitting oedema, added heart sounds, raised JVP. Radiology shows specific features (see Chapter 26).

Radiographic differentials

- Any cause of fluid in the alveoli – 'airspace disease'.
- Blood in the alveoli – traumatic contusion – should be easy to differentiate from pneumonia on clinical grounds.
- Cardiac failure – see above.
- Tumour – bronchioloalveolar carcinoma. It can be radiologically indistinguishable from pneumonia. The difference is that it does not resolve with treatment.
- Infarction – in pulmonary embolism – usually wedge shaped and may not be as extensive as infection.

Radiological features

Pneumonia can have several radiographic patterns. It can be confined to one lobe (lobar pneumonia) or be patchy and involve several lobes (bronchopneumonia). It can also cause a white-out of the hemithorax (see Chapter 9).

Fig. 8.1 is an example of both a white-out and right lower lobe pneumonia.

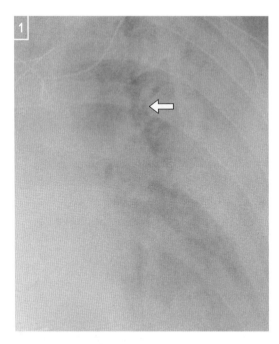

Fig. 8.1B The consolidation appears of increased density and is patchy. This is in contrast to collapses (Chapter 17) and pleural effusions (Chapter 20), which are more homogeneous. Consolidation may also contain air bronchograms (arrow). This is an exercise in understanding silhouette signs (see p. 5).

Normally, bronchi are not seen as they are effectively air dense and are superimposed on air density of the alveoli. When the alveoli fill with pus (consolidation) the air-filled bronchi are now seen, with air adjacent to water.

Silhouette signs can help localize the pneumonia and aid diagnosis.

The following are examples of pneumonia in different locations and the use of silhouette signs to localize them.

Right upper lobe pneumonia

In Fig. 8.2 the pneumonia is in the right upper lobe. It is sharply inferiorly bordered by the horizontal fissure (arrow). This patient also has an enlarged right hilum.

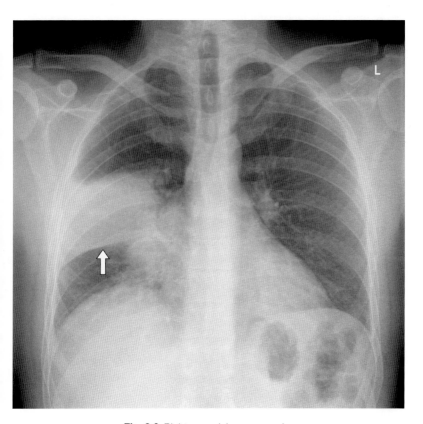

Fig. 8.2 Right upper lobe pneumonia.

Right middle lobe pneumonia

The patient shown in Fig 8.3 has consolidation in the right lower zone. There is loss of the contour of the right heart border, which implies that the consolidation abuts this edge (arrow).

The right heart border is adjacent to the right middle lobe so this is a right middle lobe pneumonia. The right hemidiaphragm is preserved (its loss would suggest lower lobe pathology).

Note the pleural effusion – a complication of pneumonia (see Chapter 20).

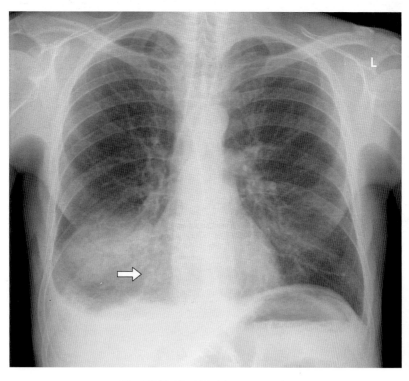

Fig. 8.3 Right middle lobe pneumonia.

Right lower lobe pneumonia

The patient shown in Fig. 8.4 also has right lower zone consolidation but the contour of the right hemidiaphragm is lost (arrow). This structure abuts the right lower lobe. Note preservation of the right heart border this time. This is a right lower lobe pneumonia.

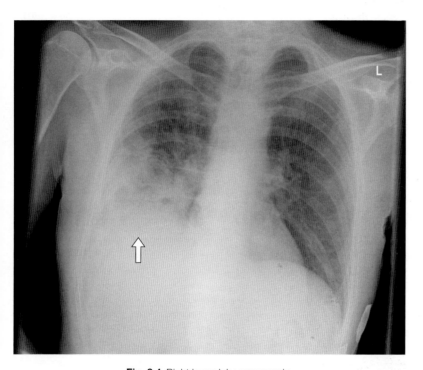

Fig. 8.4 Right lower lobe pneumonia.

Left lower lobe pneumonia

This is an important and frequently missed location for pneumonia.

In Fig. 8.5, note the increased density behind the heart and loss of the contour of the left hemidiaphragm (arrow). This is a left lower lobe pneumonia. It also affects the lingular segment of the left upper lobe (this is the equivalent of the right middle lobe) – as evidenced by loss of the contour of the left heart border.

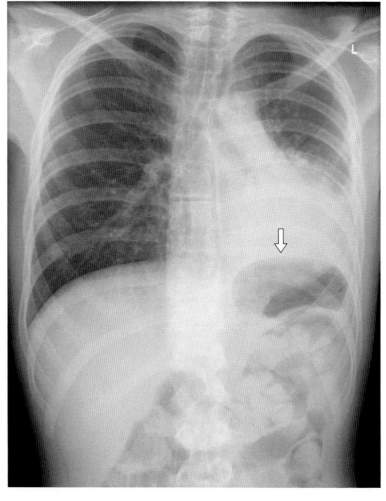

Fig. 8.5 Left lower lobe pneumonia.

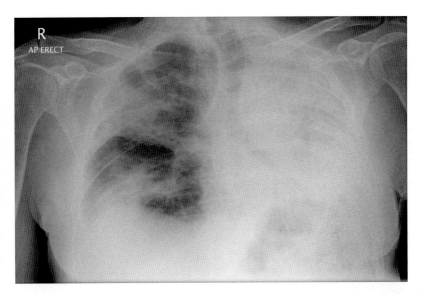

Fig. 8.6 Bronchioloalveolar carcinoma.

Bronchioloalveolar carcinoma

The patient shown in Fig. 8.6 had a proven bronchioloalveolar carcinoma. This is indistinguishable from pneumonia – but it worsened over several months and the diagnosis was eventually made by bronchoalveolar lavage.

Round pneumonia

Round pneumonia is more commonly seen in young children than adults. It is important to be aware that pneumonia can have this radiological appearance as it can simulate a mass lesion (Fig. 8.7, arrows). The border is often slightly irregular but the presence of air bronchograms may help you make the diagnosis.

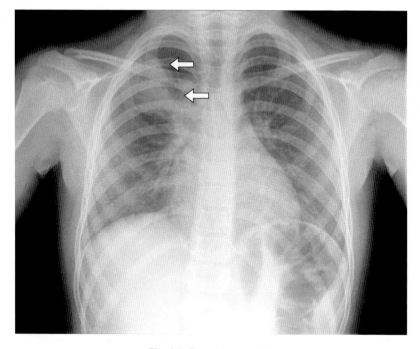

Fig. 8.7 Round pneumonia.

Important management points and further investigations
Immediate management

- Commence the patient on oxygen therapy.
- Take bloods, blood cultures and blood gases. These can help to determine severity.

Once a confident diagnosis of pneumonia has been made:

- Commence intravenous antibiotics depending on local sensitivities and the presumed cause (community-acquired pneumonia and hospital-acquired pneumonia generally require different antibiotic regimens). Most units have guidelines for the use of antibiotics in both community- and hospital-acquired pneumonia. Obtain advice from microbiology if you are unsure.

The CURB 65 score can be helpful for assessment of severity [1]. Score 1 for each of the below:

C Confusion
U Urea >7 mmol/L
R Respiratory rate >30/min
B Systolic BP <90 mmHg or diastolic BP <60 mmHg
65 Age >65.

A score of 2 or more indicates an increased risk of mortality: involve your senior early. You may need the help of the ITU.

Further management considerations

Remember that you should make sure the pneumonia has resolved. Arrange repeat radiography in 6 weeks (Royal College of Radiologists recommendation). If it has not resolved consider the possibility of tumour.

Repeated infection may also be the explanation for persistent consolidation (e.g. bronchiectasis – Chapter 13).

Further imaging

This is not usually necessary.

Reference

[1] Lim WS, van der Eerden MM, Laing R, et al. Defining community acquired pneumonia severity on presentation to hospital: an international derivation and validation study. Thorax 2003;58(5):377–82.

9 White-out hemithorax

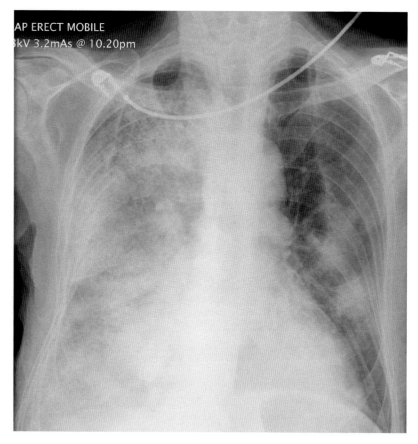

Fig. 9.1 White-out of the right hemithorax caused by a right-sided pneumonia.

Background

White-out hemithorax is an important radiological appearance because all three causes occur in unwell patients. These three causes are extensive pneumonia, collapse of the whole lung, and a massive pleural effusion.

They can be differentiated by clinical and radiological features, and by complex imaging.

Clinical features

See each separate chapter for clinical presentations:

- Pneumonia, Chapter 8
- Pleural effusion, Chapter 20
- Lobar collapses, Chapter 17.

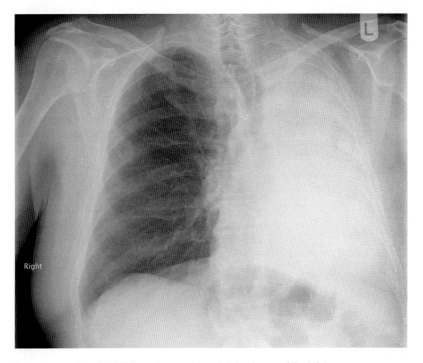

Fig. 9.2 White-out caused by a total collapse of the left lung.

Radiological features

The key to interpretation is the position of the mediastinum.

In pneumonia (Fig. 9.1), there is no loss of volume in the lung so the mediastinum and trachea remain central. The other clue in pneumonia is that the shadowing may be a little patchy and there may be air bronchograms.

In lung collapse (Fig. 9.2), there is loss of volume as the alveoli are all collapsed. The mediastinum and trachea move toward the side of the pathology. A pneumonectomy will produce the same appearance, in a well patient, usually with evidence of a thoracotomy (missing rib).

In pleural effusion (Fig. 9.3) the additional volume of the pleural fluid in addition to the lung push the mediastinum away.

Bear in mind that these three conditions may coexist. Pneumonia is a cause of effusions. A lung tumour causing a global collapse may coexist with a pleural effusion. Real life is seldom straightforward!

Remember to look at old films if these are available as they may show you the story unfolding (e.g. an effusion gradually increasing in size).

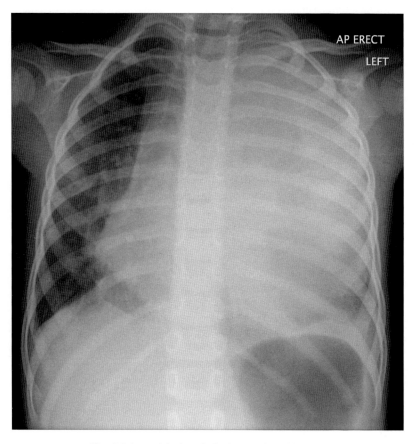

Fig. 9.3 Large left pleural effusion causing white-out.

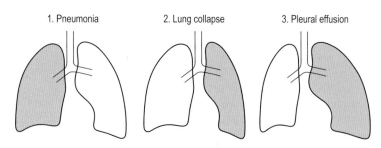

Fig. 9.4 The three causes of white-out hemithorax.

Important management points and further investigations

Immediate management

Look at old films. Correlate with the clinical presentation, paying particular attention to features such as pyrexia, productive cough and smoking history.

Further imaging

This is often necessary. A chest ultrasound will determine if there is fluid in the pleural space.

CT may be necessary in lung collapse to see if there is a central lesion present.

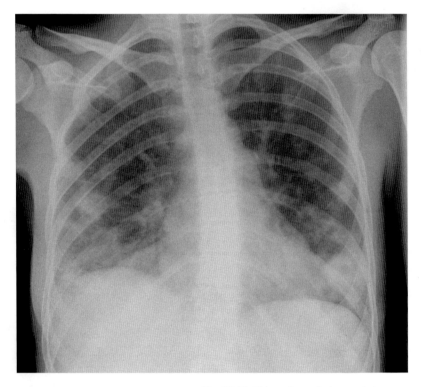

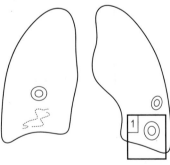

Fig. 10.1A This radiograph demonstrates several ill-defined opacities in both lungs with central cavitation. This patient was an intravenous drug abuser who had endocarditis complicated by cavitating lung abscesses.

Background

Lung abscesses are associated with a poor prognosis if not detected and treated. They are caused by lung infection; aetiologies include aspiration, pneumonia, septicaemia and endocarditis.

Clinical features

Symptoms

The symptoms are fever and productive cough with foul sputum: there may be a long history. There may also be weight loss.

Signs

Signs of endocarditis, intravenous drug abuse or dental disease may provide a clue to the aetiology. There may be associated consolidation or pleural effusion.

Differential diagnosis

Several lung processes cause cavitating masses:

- Cavitating lung metastases especially squamous primary (see Chapter 16). The clinical presentation is different.
- Connective tissue diseases such as Wegener's granulomatosis. The patient is well and often the diagnosis is made in the outpatient setting.
- TB. This condition usually affects the lung apices (see Chapter 11.)
- Empyema (see Chapter 21) – the radiological features are different.
- Cavitating carcinoma of the lung (see Chapter 15) – again the history should be different.

Radiological features

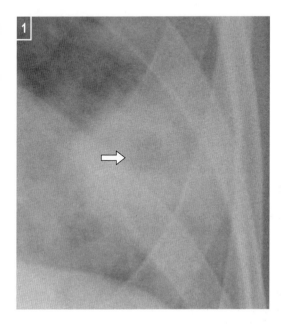

Fig. 10.1B Lung abscesses are usually ill-defined and are initially thick-walled and become more thin-walled as central necrosis progresses. They can be single or multiple. Cavitation is the hallmark, as demonstrated by a central lucent area (arrow), but early abscesses may not cavitate. Larger abscesses may contain an air–fluid level on an erect CXR. They may coexist with a pleural effusion or areas of consolidation.

Differentials: Cavitating lung metastases generally have a better-defined edge, as do vasculitic processes such as Wegener's granulomatosis.

Important management points and further investigations

Immediate management

Oxygen therapy and prompt intravenous antibiotics are important and the latter improve survival.

Inform your senior.

Further management considerations

Seek the cause. The diagnosis may not be easy and further imaging may be needed.

Involve a respiratory physician in complicated or refractory cases, or those where the diagnosis is in doubt.

Further imaging

- Serial follow-up x-rays.
- CT scan may be helpful if the diagnosis is in doubt.

11 Tuberculosis (TB)

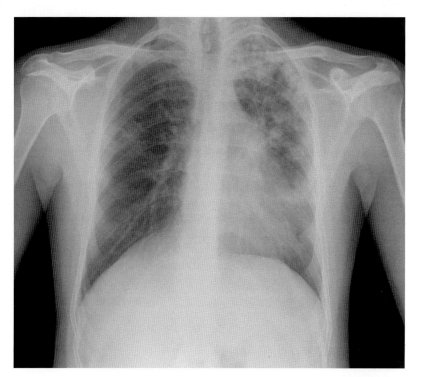

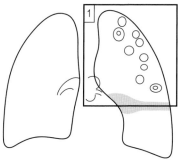

Fig. 11.1A This radiograph demonstrates an area of cavitating consolidation at the left apex. Appearance are typical of active TB.

Background

TB is transmitted by the airborne route and active TB is highly infectious. It is caused by acid-fast bacilli. Signs of old TB can often be seen on radiographs as calcified densities at the lung apices, often in elderly patients, but active TB is a condition which needs to be addressed urgently.

Pulmonary involvement is most common but it can also affect most organ systems (bones, urinary tract, GI tract).

TB is commoner in immunosuppressed patients, particularly those with HIV.

Clinical features
Symptoms

The main symptoms are cough, haemoptysis, fever, night sweats, anorexia and weight loss (active TB). There may be a history of immunosuppression. The patient's ethnicity (Asian) may be an important clue to diagnosis. Active TB can be asymptomatic.

Signs

These include lymphadenopathy (cervical), signs of consolidation, cachexia, pyrexia and hypoxia.

Radiological features

Consolidation suggests active TB.

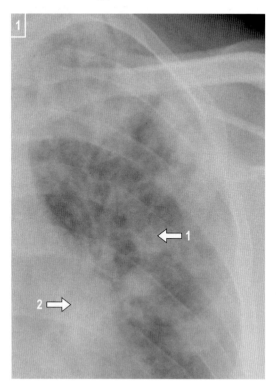

Fig. 11.1B Cavitation is an important hallmark of this condition (arrow 1). Look for a central lucent area within an area of consolidation. However, it can be difficult to distinguish true cavitation from opacity with adjacent normal lung. Hilar and/or mediastinal lymphadenopathy may be present – look for enlarged hila (arrow 2) and abnormal paratracheal convexity (not shown here). A pleural effusion may be present in active TB (see Chapter 20). Look for a calcified Ghon focus. This is the primary site of infection and is usually situated in the mid-zones. See also next chapter on miliary TB.

The differential diagnoses of cavitating lesions include non-TB abscesses (Chapter 10), cavitating tumours (primary or metastases; Chapter 15 & 16) and more rarely granulomatoses.

Old TB has the appearance of fibrosis and scarring at the apices with loss of apical lung volume (hila pulled upwards).

Important management points and further investigations

Immediate management

- Inform your senior if this diagnosis is suspected. Management of such cases is complex.
- Isolate the patient in a side room with barrier nursing.
- Involve the infectious diseases team early.
- This diagnosis can be difficult to make on a plain radiograph: consider obtaining the help of a radiologist.

Further management considerations

Confirmation by the microbiologist with sputum microscopy and Ziehl–Neelsen staining is advised. Acid-fast bacilli are seen. This is a quick test to do in practice.

Tuberculin skin testing can be used to supplement microbiology and radiology. A negative test does not necessarily exclude TB.

Patients with TB should be promptly started on quadruple therapy (rifampicin, isoniazid, pyrazinamide, ethambutol: mnemonic 'RIPE'), under the guidance of an infectious diseases team. This reduces infectivity.

Active TB is highly contagious, so if it is diagnosed, the occupational health department should be informed and contact tracing carried out. TB is a notifiable disease and this is a legal obligation.

Further imaging

Further imaging is not indicated. The diagnosis is made using a combination of plain radiography and appropriate clinical and microbiological indices as described above.

12 | Miliary TB

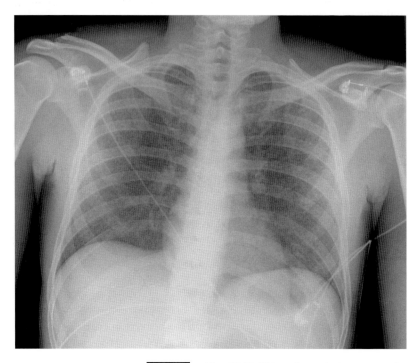

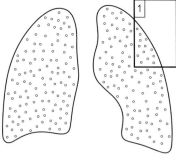

Fig. 12.1A This radiograph shows several tiny nodules scattered evenly throughout the entirety of the lungs. This patient has miliary TB.

Background

See Chapter 11.

Miliary TB is caused by haematogenous dissemination of TB bacteria and can occur during primary TB infection or several years after primary infection. Miliary TB may be seeded throughout the body and the appearances on the CXR are due to multiple caseating granulomas.

If not diagnosed and treated it is fatal.

Clinical features

These can be non-specific, underlining the importance of correctly interpreting the radiology.

Symptoms

Symptoms include cough and fever, weight loss and headache (meningeal/ brain involvement). Onset can be over days.

Signs

The patient is unwell; lymphadenopathy or hepatosplenomegaly may also be present.

Differential diagnosis

Miliary TB is the only condition with this radiographic appearance in an acutely unwell patient.

Several other conditions have the same appearance:

- In a patient with a relevant primary tumour, miliary metastases can have the same appearance – thyroid, pancreas, breast and melanoma primaries can cause this appearance.
- Sarcoidosis can also have the same appearance but the patient will be well.
- Silicosis causes tiny nodules, but with a predilection for the lung apices.

Radiological features

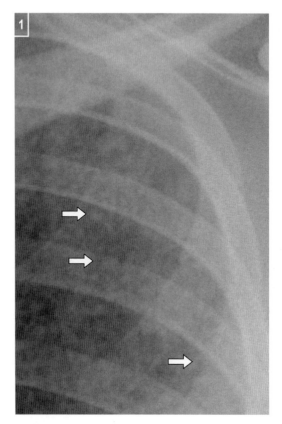

Fig. 12.1B Miliary TB is characterized by several tiny nodules evenly distributed throughout the lungs (arrows). There are numerous tiny nodules scattered throughout this close-up. Nodules are of soft tissue density in the 1–5 mm range.

Look for all the signs of primary TB – see Chapter 11.

Important management points and further investigations

Immediate management

Management is the same as for primary TB but these patients are more ill and require urgent treatment.

Further imaging

CT is more sensitive for diagnosis of miliary nodules.

13 | Bronchiectasis

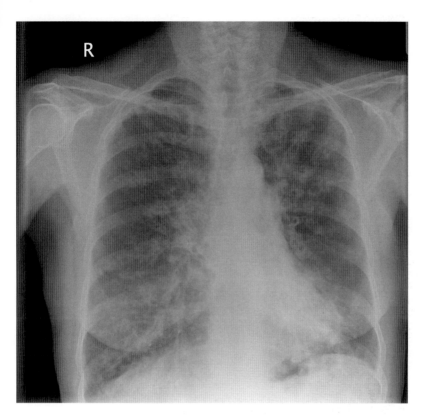

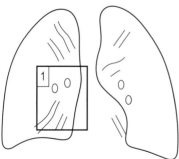

Fig. 13.1 This patient has bronchiectasis in a central distribution.

Background

Bronchiectasis refers to permanent dilatation of bronchi and bronchioles. This leads to recurrent chest infections and sputum production. The condition can affect both children and adults. Causes may be post-infective (measles, pneumonia, TB – upper lobes primarily affected), congenital (cystic fibrosis, Kartagener's), or due to several rarer factors.

Clinical features

Symptoms

The main symptoms are chronic cough and sputum production, haemoptysis and weight loss.

Signs

- Signs of chest infection
- Persistent coarse crepitations in between acute infective exacerbations.

The diagnosis of bronchiectasis is not an emergency per se, but patients may present acutely to a medical ward with symptoms related to bronchiectasis.

Radiological features

Remember that plain films are not very sensitive early in this condition and that high-resolution CT is the gold standard. But, as is often the case, the plain film findings may point you in the right direction in an unwell patient presenting with some of the above clinical features.

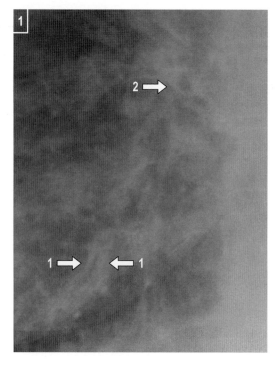

Fig. 13.2 The signs of bronchiectasis relate to thick-walled dilated bronchi. Think of these when interpreting the film. Bronchi imaged side-on appear as 'tramline shadows' which relate to a thickened dilated bronchus side-on (arrows 1). Central bronchi which are imaged en face, or coming toward the viewer, are ring shaped and form ring shadows (arrow 2). This is a similar principle to the peribronchial cuffing seen in cardiac failure (see Ch. 26, p. 133).

Remember that superadded infection can obscure these findings, and in the patient with pneumonia, bronchiectasis can be the underlying cause. Look at old films and take further radiographs after suitable treatment.

Important management points and further investigations

Immediate management

No immediate action is necessarily required although this finding may be very relevant in an unwell patient with respiratory symptoms. Treat infection if it is present. Chest physiotherapy is helpful in this group of patients.

Further imaging

High-resolution CT is the most sensitive modality for accurate diagnosis.

14 Chronic obstructive pulmonary disease (COPD)

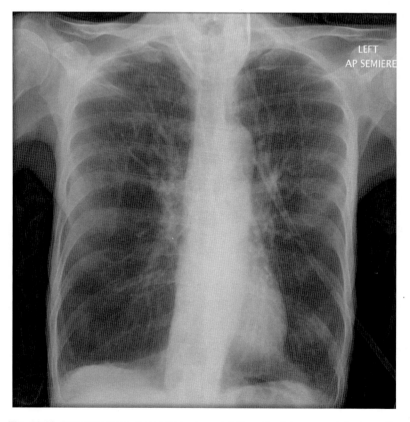

Fig. 14.1A This radiograph demonstrates hyperinflation of both lungs, a relatively small cardiac shadow and flattened hemidiaphragms in keeping with COPD.

Background

COPD refers to the combination of chronic bronchitis and emphysema. It is a very common condition, and smoking is the commonest cause.

This is not intended to be an exhaustive account of this very large topic, rather an account of the plain film findings in this condition.

The on-call doctor (usually medicine or A&E) will commonly admit these patients with an infective exacerbation causing wheezing and breathlessness.

Clinical features

Symptoms

- Long history of worsening breathlessness
- Symptoms of infection/wheezing in infective exacerbations.

Signs

- Hyperresonant barrel chest
- Wheezing
- Signs of right heart failure in cor pulmonale.

Differential diagnosis

Asthma – which occurs in non-smokers, often of a younger age. The key difference is that people with asthma are not breathless between attacks.

Radiological features

This is not a diagnosis made on the CXR but features on the CXR can help make the diagnosis.

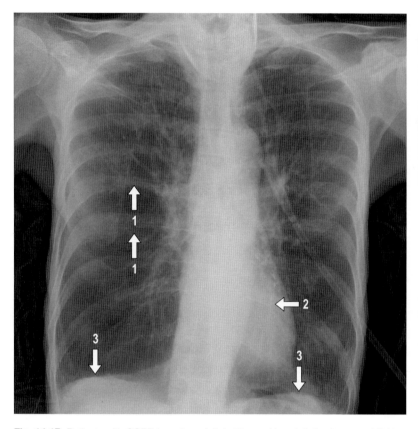

Fig. 14.1B Patients with COPD have hyperinflated lungs. Hyperinflation is present if 11 or more posterior ribs (arrows 1) are visualized. Very occasionally a normal young patient achieves this by making an excellent inspiration. The hyperinflated lungs compress the heart, making the cardiac silhouette look rather small (arrow 2). The hemidiaphragms are also pushed down and flattened (arrows 3). Central lung markings may appear more prominent than in a non-smoker without COPD.

Remember to look for a pneumothorax – a recognized associated complication of COPD (see Chapter 18).

The radiograph may demonstrate focal consolidation (see Chapter 8).

Important management points and further investigations

Immediate management

Arterial blood gas analysis will give an indication of severity.

Careful oxygen therapy is important; 100% oxygen carries the theoretical risk of depressing the respiratory hypercapnic drive to breathe – 28% oxygen is usually given.

Treatment with antibiotics, nebulizers and steroids is indicated for infective exacerbations.

Further imaging

Further imaging is not usually indicated.

Emphysematous change is better seen on CT than plain films, often as an incidental finding. CT is not normally performed to diagnose COPD.

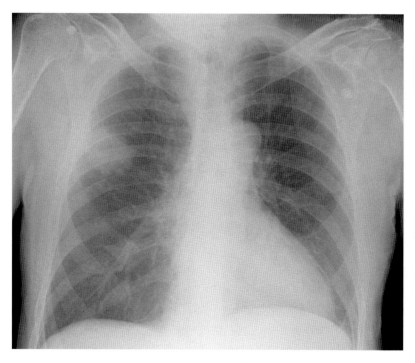

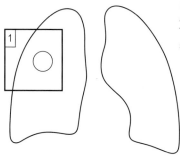

Fig. 15.1A This patient has a rounded irregular abnormality in the right mid-zone peripherally. This is a solitary pulmonary nodule, with subsequent diagnosis of lung cancer.

Background

The solitary pulmonary nodule may be encountered in the patient presenting acutely, or in the outpatient setting, and detecting a malignant pulmonary nodule is important for patient management. The differential diagnosis of a solitary nodule on a CXR is wide but the possibility of malignancy should always be considered.

- Is the patient a smoker and at risk?
- Does the patient have a known malignancy to make a metastasis a possibility?

This abnormality may be encountered by any doctor who evaluates CXRs and should be sought on every CXR.

Differential diagnosis

Common causes to be considered are:
- primary tumour (malignant) – lung carcinoma
- primary tumour (benign) – adenoma/hamartoma
- secondary tumour (metastasis)
- granuloma (calcified)
- abscess (see Chapter 10)
- arteriovenous malformation (often has vessels entering and leaving it – CT can confirm).

There are many rarer causes.

Radiological features

The features shown in Fig. 15.1B raise the possibility of malignancy, but it is often very difficult to be confident of malignancy on a plain film and the help of a radiologist should be sought.

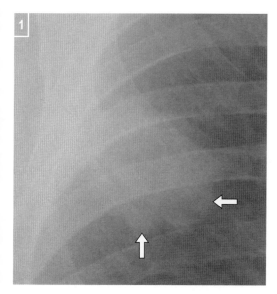

Fig. 15.1B Malignant nodules often have irregular, ill-defined or spiculated borders (arrows). This is in contrast with benign nodules which are often well defined and calcified.

Look at old x-rays – if the nodule has grown or is new the chance of malignancy is higher. If it has been there for 10 years it is almost certainly benign.

Your safety net with these films is that they will be reported by a radiologist and hopefully the abnormality spotted then, but it is best to make the diagnosis early before discharging the patient.

Look for rib metastases and an enlarged hilum or mediastinum, which would increase suspicion of malignancy. Remember to hunt for lung tumours in your review areas – the right apex is a common site. This is also a site with many composite shadows where tumours are often missed.

Also look behind the heart – many cancers are missed here.

Lung cancers are most commonly seen at the hilum. Hilar enlargement or increased density should be evaluated further. Old films are useful in assessment to see if any change has occurred.

Important management points and further investigations
Immediate management

The patient is not necessarily at immediate risk but the finding might indicate why they are unwell.

Further management considerations

Patient will often require a CT scan for further characterisation and staging.

A respiratory referral and discussion at the respiratory MDT will help plan further management.

Further reading

Gaude GS, Pinto MJ. Evaluation of solitary pulmonary nodule. J Postgrad Med 1995;41:56–9.

16 Lung metastases – multiple pulmonary nodules

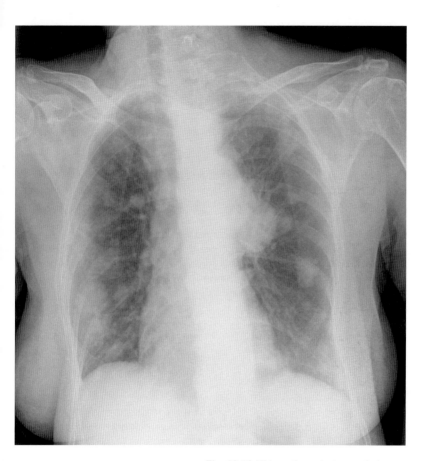

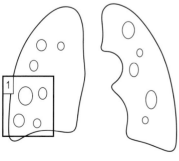

Fig. 16.1A This radiograph demonstrates several round soft tissue nodules of varying sizes. This patient has multiple lung metastases.

Background

This is an appearance that any doctor interpreting chest radiographs may encounter, and may be seen on-call as well as in the outpatient clinic. It is important to make an accurate diagnosis and correctly manage the patient as there is a considerable differential diagnosis.

In the patient whose radiograph demonstrates several rounded soft tissue lesions the diagnosis of metastases should be considered, particularly if the patient has a known primary cancer.

The patient may also have symptoms relating to lung metastases, such as breathlessness and weight loss.

Differential diagnosis

Most causes of solitary pulmonary nodules (Chapter 15) can also cause multiple nodules.

The differential diagnosis includes:

- lung metastases
- lung abscesses (Chapter 10): these patients are usually unwell
- multiple granulomas – should be stable in appearance on old films, and are calcified
- multiple arteriovenous malformations (AVMs) – these classically have an afferent and efferent vessel connecting them to the ipsilateral hilum
- granulomatous diseases, such as Wegener's granulomatosis – these often cavitate.

There are several other causes.

Radiological features

As with the solitary pulmonary nodule, previous x-rays are very important for diagnosis. Acute processes such as abscesses appear very quickly over days. Metastases grow in size over months depending on the primary and may be evident on old films. Chronic processes such as granulomas stay constant for years.

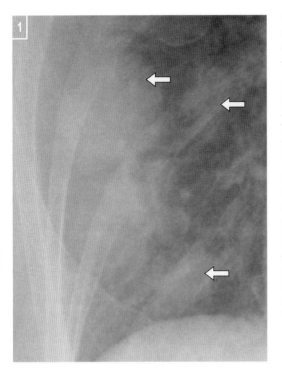

Fig. 16.1B Well-defined, rounded soft tissue masses in the lungs (arrows). These are pulmonary metastases.

Lung metastases usually have well-defined edges and can be distinguished from areas of consolidation as they are generally quite homogeneous in density.

Lung metastases can be very subtle on CXRs and their size can vary considerably. They can be tiny or quite large – 'cannonball metastases'. They can also cavitate centrally (cf. lung abscess, Chapter 10); this most commonly occurs in squamous tumours.

Lung metastases are generally randomly distributed throughout the lungs and do not have a predilection for any particular zone.

Look for other clues as to the diagnosis, such as missing ribs (metastases), a thoracotomy, mastectomy, or a mass at the hilum, which may represent a bronchogenic primary.

Important management points and further investigations

Immediate management

These patients are not necessarily at any immediate risk. This diagnosis will obviously impact considerably on their further management.

Further imaging

The finding of lung metastases will often prompt the hunt for a primary.

Start the search clinically – e.g. examine for breast lumps or perform a rectal examination to look for a rectal/prostatic tumour.

Imaging with CT of the chest, abdomen and pelvis is often performed to locate a primary in patients in whom clinical examination and basic investigations are not forthcoming. There is some debate regarding the clinical benefit of determining a primary site in patients with disseminated metastases and systemic symptoms, so further imaging should be performed in the context of the patient's condition.

17 Lobar collapses

Background

Collapse of the five lung lobes (right upper, middle and lower, left upper and lower) produces characteristic appearances on a CXR. Interpretation requires a good knowledge of lobar anatomy and of silhouette signs (see Page 5).

Lobar collapses are important as they are a common presentation of bronchial carcinoma (see Chapter 15). Other causes of lobar collapse include any process that obstructs a main bronchus, including mucus plugging in asthmatics and postoperative patients, foreign bodies and ET tubes (these usually cause complete collapse; see Chapter 2).

General radiological features common to all collapses

- A radiological hallmark of all collapses is **loss of lung volume on the affected side**, which worsens in chronic collapse – if the collapse is acute there may be no loss of volume.
- The ribs may come closer together when volume is lost on one side.
- Volume loss may also result in a tented raised hemidiaphragm on the side of the collapse.
- There may be mediastinal shift toward the collapsed side.
- Look for a mass at the hilum, which would increase suspicion of a tumour as the cause. However, a tumour may be present and not seen due to the collapse and any new unexplained collapse warrants further imaging/investigation.
- The remainder of the lung on the side of the collapse may be more lucent than that on the opposite side, with a decreased vessel count.

Remember to use the silhouette sign to your advantage.

A collapsed lobe is of increased density. Remember that edges are only seen on films if two structures of different density are next to each other. In lung collapse a lobe effectively becomes water/soft tissue dense. So if an edge you would expect to see disappears this might help you determine which lobe is collapsed.

For example, in left lower lobe collapse, the left lower lobe is adjacent to the left hemidiaphragm. When this lobe collapses the contour of the left hemidiaphragm is no longer seen.

Collapsed lung is generally homogeneous in density – with no air bronchograms seen.

Background anatomy

A sound knowledge of lobar anatomy is vital for understanding of collapse.

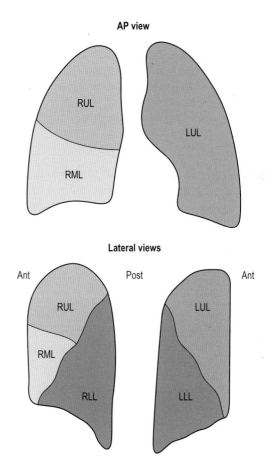

AP view

Lateral views

Right upper lobe collapse

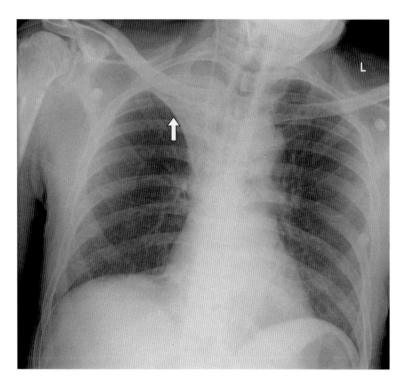

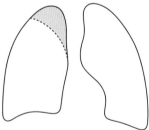

Fig. 17.1 Right upper lobe collapse. Note the right-sided central line.

In right upper lobe collapse, the lobe collapses upwards.

The collapsed lobe is inferiorly bounded by the horizontal fissure so look for increased opacification at the right apex, inferiorly bounded by the straight or superiorly convex line of the horizontal fissure, which has been pulled upwards (Fig. 17.1, arrow).

Look for general signs of collapse on this side as above.

Right middle lobe collapse

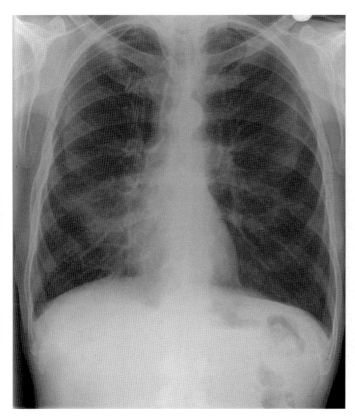

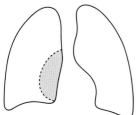

Fig. 17.2 Right middle lobe collapse.

Right middle lobe collapse is one of the most difficult to diagnose as it can be very subtle. The collapse has the appearance of increased opacification adjacent to the right heart border. The silhouette sign is particularly helpful here as loss of the right heart border confirms the position of the pathology. The appearance can be indistinguishable from a right middle lobe pneumonia. A lateral film may be helpful to confirm the diagnosis.

87

Right lower lobe collapse

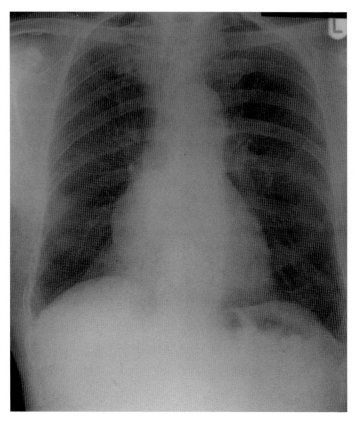

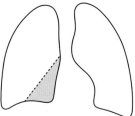

Fig. 17.3 Right lower lobe collapse.

The right lower lobe collapses inferoposteriorly. Look for the straight edge of the oblique fissure.

The right hemidiaphragm is lost (medially in Fig. 17.3), and the right heart border preserved.

Left upper lobe collapse

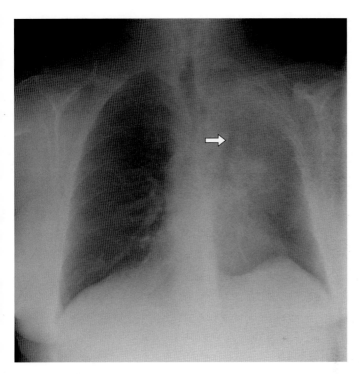

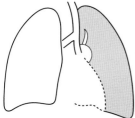

Fig. 17.4 Left upper lobe collapse.

The left upper lobe is anterior in location, occupying the whole anterior part of the left hemithorax. It collapses forwards, thus causing opacity over the whole left hemithorax. There are no sharp demarcating edges. The opacity is classically 'veil-like'. The left lower lobe expands upwards to occupy the space and can extend as high as adjacent to the aortic knuckle, this appearance is seen on this radiograph and is called the luftsichel sign (Fig. 17.4, arrow). Note in Fig. 17.4 the marked left-sided volume loss and tenting of the hemidiaphragm, as well as tracheal deviation toward the collapse. It is just possible to make out a mass at the left hilum, which is the cause for this appearance.

Left lower lobe collapse

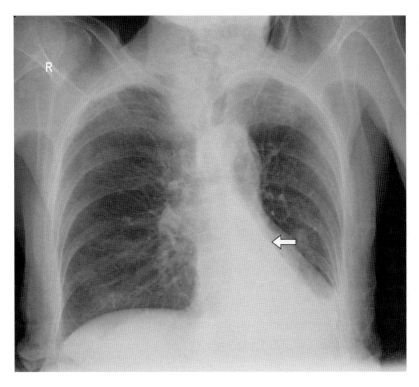

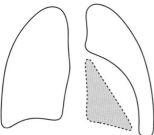

Fig. 17.5 Left lower lobe collapse (see overleaf).

The left lower lobe collapses posteromedially and this is a mirror image of the right lower lobe collapse.

It underlines the importance of looking behind the heart as a review area as this appearance can be very subtle. It can have the appearance of a sail behind the heart, with a triangle of increased density, laterally bounded by a straight edge, which is the oblique fissure (Fig. 17.5, arrow).

See also the chapter on white out hemithorax, which discusses complete lung collapse (Chapter 9).

Further management and imaging

The finding of a new or unexplained lobar collapse should raise concern about an underlying bronchial carcinoma.

In the first instance, a CT scan with contrast of the thorax and liver should be performed. Bronchoscopy should be considered, and the patient should be referred to the lung multidisciplinary team for prompt management.

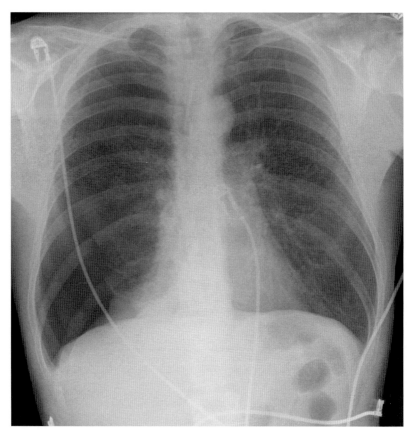

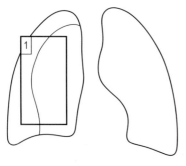

Fig. 18.1A This erect radiograph shows a right-sided simple pneumothorax.

Background

Causes

- Spontaneous (in tall males, Marfan syndrome)
- Secondary to chronic lung disease – asthma/COPD
- Iatrogenic: central line insertion (see Ch. 3), lung biopsy, mechanical ventilation
- Infections: certain pneumonias (Klebsiella, TB, staphylococcal)
- Trauma.

Types of pneumothorax

- Simple pneumothorax – air in the pleural space.
- Open pneumothorax – an open communication between the outside world and the pleural cavity. This is a medical emergency which is often caused by penetrating trauma. Sealing the connection between the outside world and the pneumothorax converts it to a closed pneumothorax.
- Tension pneumothorax – requires immediate treatment as it is a life-threatening condition, which can lead to cardiovascular collapse. Tension pneumothorax is caused by a 'one-way valve' communication between the lung and pleura or outside world and pleura which allows air into but not out of the pleural cavity. This causes rapid build-up of air, which compresses adjacent vascular structures such as the superior vena cava. This reduces venous return to the heart and thus rapidly leads to cardiac arrest.

Tension pneumothorax is a **clinical diagnosis**. By the time a CXR has been arranged, the patient may be dead. If suspected it must be treated immediately. (See Figs 18.6–18.8.)

Clinical features

Symptoms

- Sudden onset chest pain on the side of the pneumothorax, often pleuritic
- Dyspnoea (worsening in tension pneumothorax).

Signs

- Hyperresonance on the side of the pneumothorax
- Tracheal shift away from the side of the pneumothorax
- Hyperexpansion of the chest
- Tachypnoea and tachycardia
- Raised JVP
- Hypotension
- Pulsus paradoxus.

Signs of tension pneumothorax are relatively non-specific but always consider the clinical context and think of this diagnosis in the **deteriorating** patient.

Radiological features

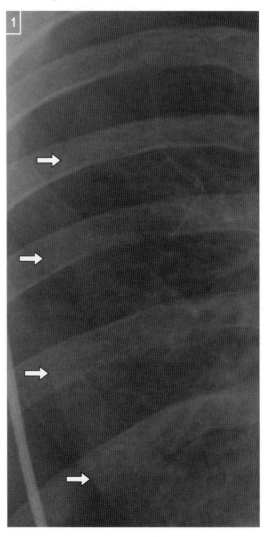

Fig. 18.1B On an erect film, the signs of pneumothorax are as follows:

In the presence of a pneumothorax, there is air in the pleural space and the lung collapses down so its edge is seen (arrows).

No normal lung markings are seen lateral to the lung edge.

Normal lung markings are seen medial to the lung edge.

A small pneumothorax can be very subtle, look at the lung apex as this is often where they start.

There are several mimics of pneumothorax (see below).

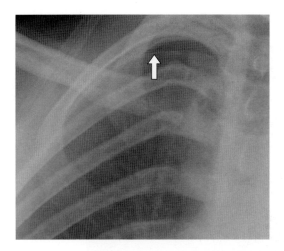

Fig. 18.2 Apical pneumothorax – different patient. The apex is a difficult part of the lung field to analyse as there are many overlapping outlines from the bones. This is a subtle pneumothorax.

The lung edge can be seen between the second and third interspaces (arrow). As above, there are no vascular markings beyond the lung edge.

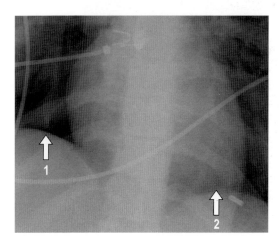

Fig. 18.3 Supine pneumothorax. Interpretation of the supine patient with a pneumothorax can be difficult. Trauma patients may be immobilized on a board so a supine portable film has to be taken (see p. 3). The air in the pleural space can track anteriorly so that a lung edge is not seen. Look for a very sharply defined mediastinal and medial diaphragmatic contour – it is well defined because air, which is of a different density, is adjacent to it. Here, the right heart border and right medial hemidiaphragm are sharply outlined (arrow 1), while the left heart border and hemidiaphragm are normal (arrow 2).

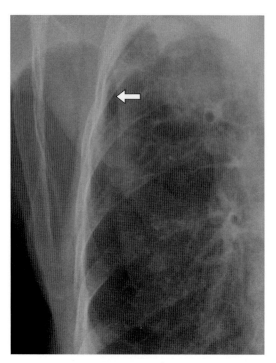

Fig. 18.4 Skin fold mimicking pneumothorax. A skin fold can cause a vertical line, which can simulate the lung edge (arrow). However, there will be lung markings lateral to the line. Sometimes the line will extend outside the hemithorax.

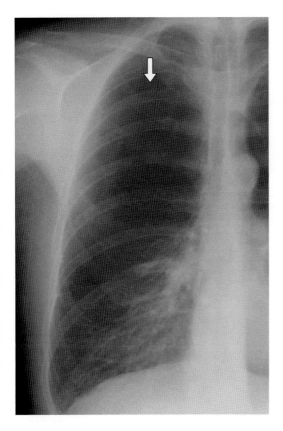

Fig. 18.5 In patients with end-stage emphysema a large bulla can simulate a pneumothorax. These can be very difficult to differentiate from a pneumothorax as a peripherally situated bulla will not contain lung markings (arrow). The problem is compounded by the fact that patients with emphysema can suffer pneumothoraces as a complication of their disease. Inserting a chest drain into a bulla is effectively the same as inserting the drain into the lung – not desirable – and can result in a bronchopleural fistula.

CT may be required to differentiate between a large bulla and pneumothorax.

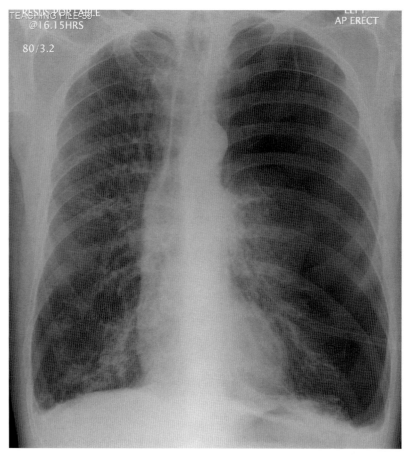

TEACHING FILE 33
@16.15HRS

80/3.2

LEFT
AP ERECT

Fig. 18.6 This patient has a left pneumothorax. However, there are signs of **tension:** the left hemidiaphragm is flattened and the mediastinum pushed to the right.

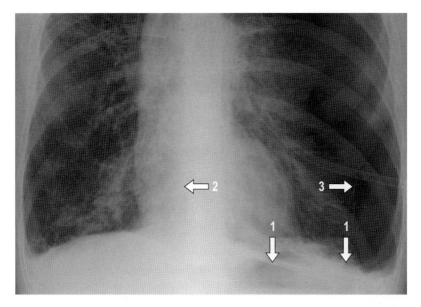

Fig. 18.7 Tension pneumothorax. The left hemidiaphragm is flattened (arrows 1) and the mediastinum shifted to the right (arrow 2). The lung edge with no markings beyond it can again be seen (arrow 3). These are the signs of a tension pneumothorax.

Important management points and further investigations
Immediate management
Your first priority is to establish if there are any signs of tension.

If a tension pneumothorax is suspected in a patient who is deteriorating, **you do not have time to perform chest radiography.** Get senior help immediately.

Ensure the airway is patent, particularly in the setting of trauma.

Place the patient on 100% oxygen; continuous saturation monitoring and frequent observations, preferably in a high dependency environment (such as the resuscitation room in A&E), are recommended. Consider arterial blood gas analysis.

Correct management is **immediate** decompression by inserting a large-bore cannula into the second intercostal space in the mid-clavicular line. A hiss of air through the cannula will confirm this diagnosis. This should be followed by insertion of a chest drain.

In the **stable** patient, who has undergone senior review, expedient portable chest radiography can be considered if the diagnosis is unclear.

It is important to recognize the signs of tension pneumothorax on a plain film, as it may be an unexpected finding in a rapidly deteriorating patient that requires the doctor to initiate the correct management immediately. The reporting radiologist should phone the clinician if the signs of tension are there but by this time it may be too late.

For traumatic and secondary pneumothorax, insertion of a chest drain should be considered.

Aspiration and observation may be sufficient for management of simple pneumothorax.

Further management considerations

Patients with a pneumothorax usually require admission to the ward.

Pleurodesis can be considered to prevent recurrence in simple pneumothoraces (under the direction of a specialist).

Further imaging

This is not necessarily indicated.

In the multiply injured trauma patient, CT of the thorax and any other sites of suspected injury should be considered.

CT can also be useful if a large bulla is suspected.

Neonatal pneumothorax

Neonatal pneumothorax can be spontaneous or iatrogenic, secondary to assisted ventilation. It is associated with several respiratory conditions, such as respiratory distress syndrome, meconium aspiration and pneumonia.

The neonate may be asymptomatic, or present with respiratory distress. Signs are similar to those in adults with hyperresonance on the affected side and tracheal deviation away from the pneumothorax. The affected side may transilluminate better than the normal side.

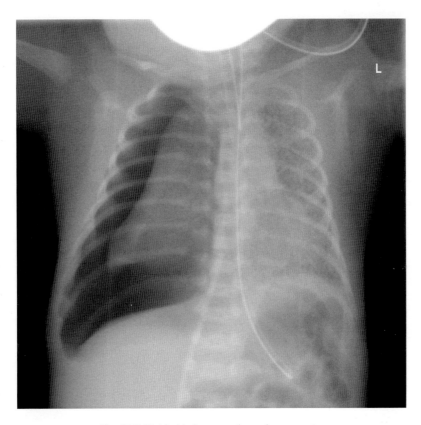

Fig. 18.8 Right-sided pneumothorax in a neonate.

Fig. 18.8 demonstrates a right-sided tension pneumothorax in a neonate. In a ventilated neonate, pneumothorax is most often of tension type. There is air in the pleural space, shift of the mediastinum to the left and a deep sulcus sign on the right – the diaphragm is pushed downwards.

A commoner appearance of a pneumothorax in a neonate on a chest radiograph, which is taken supine, is the deep sulcus sign on its own, with a sharply demarcated mediastinal and cardiac border. A lung edge is often not seen.

The patient in Fig. 18.8 requires decompression and an urgent chest drain. Note the appropriately positioned NG tube.

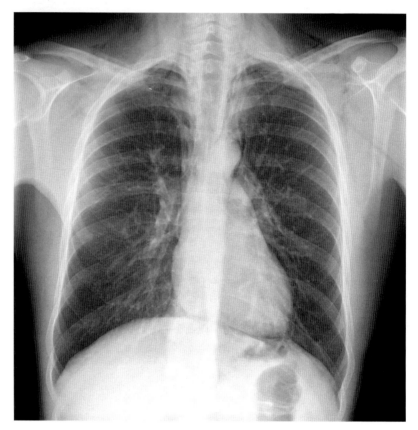

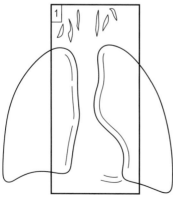

Fig. 19.1A This patient has extensive pneumomediastinum. (With thanks to Dr Godfrey Chatora for providing this radiograph.)

Background

Pneumomediastinum refers to air in the mediastinal cavity. There are several causes including asthma, trauma and Boerhaave syndrome. It can also occur spontaneously.

Boerhaave syndrome refers to rupture of the oesophagus, most often caused by forceful vomiting, and is a diagnosis which should always be thought about as it carries a high mortality (50%). Prompt diagnosis and treatment is required to increase the patient's chance of survival.

Pneumomediastinum can coexist with pneumothorax and pneumoperitoneum due to gas tracking into other body compartments.

Clinical features

Symptoms

- Often none, other than those relating to the predisposing cause
- Retrosternal chest pain
- Dysphagia and fever in Boerhaave syndrome.

Seek to elicit a relevant clinical setting, e.g. asthma, trauma, vomiting.

Signs

Subcutaneous emphysema may be present.

A crackling sound may be heard in the mediastinum on auscultation.

Differential diagnosis

The radiological appearance is pathognomonic.

Radiological features

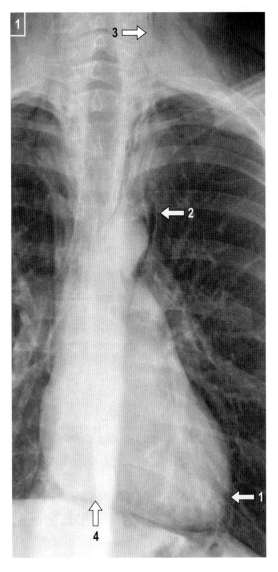

Fig. 19.1B Air is seen surrounding the mediastinum, around the heart (arrow 1) and surrounding the upper mediastinal structures such as the aortic knuckle (arrow 2).

Air may also be seen tracking into the soft tissues of the neck (arrow 3).

Look for a coexistent pneumothorax (see Chapter 18).

The left and right diaphragmatic outlines are not usually continuous. In pneumopericardium a 'continuous diaphragm sign' may be seen linking the diaphragmatic contours. This is caused by air in the pericardium (arrow 4). This does not occur in pneumomediastinum alone as the pericardium is attached to the central tendon of the diaphragm. The continuous diaphragm sign may also be seen in pneumoperitoneum (see Chapter 27).

A left-sided pleural effusion in the correct clinical setting raises the possibility of Boerhaave syndrome.

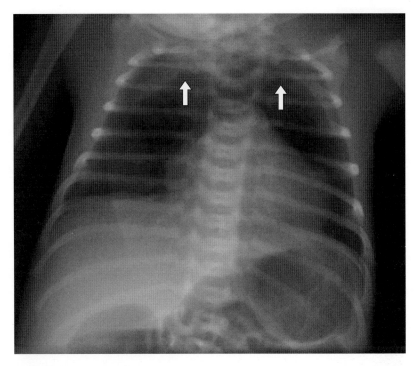

Fig. 19.2 'Spinnaker' sail sign of pneumomediastinum in an infant. The air in the mediastinum pushes up the thymus gland (arrows) causing the appearance of a spinnaker sail. This may be the only sign in this age group.

Important management points and further investigations

Immediate management

Management depends on the cause.

Supportive measures such as oxygen administration and intravenous fluid should be considered.

Senior opinion should be sought promptly in suspected Boerhaave syndrome as this condition can rapidly be lethal and generally requires an operation for correction.

Spontaneous pneumomediastinum can be managed conservatively.

Further imaging

A contrast swallow examination may be helpful for diagnosis of Boerhaave syndrome. CT is more sensitive than chest radiography for diagnosis of pneumomediastinum but is not indicated if pneumomediastinum is obvious on CXR.

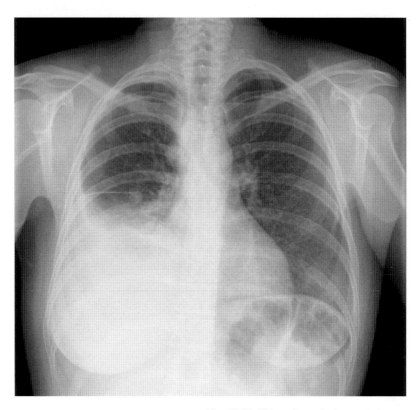

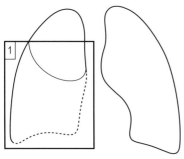

Fig. 20.1A This radiograph demonstrates a moderate right pleural effusion, with a meniscus at its upper aspect, and loss of the contour of the right hemidiaphragm.

Background

Pleural effusion refers to a collection of fluid in the pleural space. There are several causes:

- Exudates (high protein) – causes include infection and malignancy.
- Transudates (low protein) – causes include cardiac, renal and hepatic failure, pancreatitis, etc.
- Empyema – pus in the pleural space – is a type of pleural effusion – (see Chapter 21).

This is an important appearance to be aware of, as a pleural effusion can be a sign of underlying disease and may be responsible for patient symptoms such as shortness of breath. The presence of an effusion should prompt a search for an underlying cause.

Radiological features

Diagnosis is not always straightforward, as these cases illustrate.

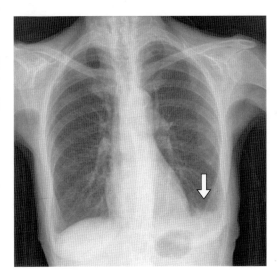

Fig. 20.2 This different patient has a small pleural effusion (arrow). The earliest sign of an effusion is blunting of the costophrenic angle. This does not necessarily mean that the effusion is small – 500 ml can collect beneath the hemidiaphragm on an erect film before anything is seen at all. The pleural space surrounds the lung and fluid sinks to the bottom. This may help in understanding the progression in appearances as the effusion gets bigger.

This is an erect film.

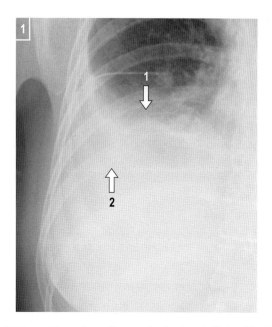

Fig. 20.1B A close-up of the patient with a moderate pleural effusion (Fig. 20.1A). The effusion has a meniscus – a concave upper border (arrow 1). The right hemithorax is filling with fluid in the pleural space which collects dependently, pushing the lung base up.

Note that the pleural space collection is of homogeneous density, as you might expect from a fluid collection, with no air bronchograms and no patchiness as is seen in airspace shadowing (see Chapter 8). The contour of the right hemidiaphragm is lost too as the fluid sits on top of it and is of the same density; hence the edge is lost – a silhouette sign (arrow 2) – (see p. 5).

This is also an erect film.

A pleural effusion can become sufficiently large that it occupies the whole hemithorax, thus producing a 'white-out', shifting the normally central heart and mediastinal structures to the opposite side (see Chapter 9).

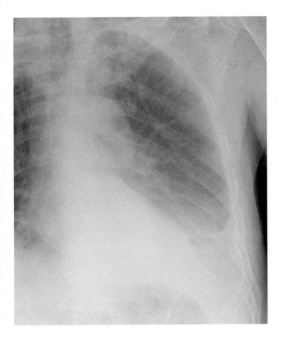

Fig. 20.3 Supine pleural effusion – different patient. The appearance of the effusion changes, as can be predicted by anatomy – if the patient is lying on their back, the pleural fluid now collects in the posterior pleura as well as inferiorly.

The superior margin of the fluid is now less well defined and the effusion takes on a hazy quality through which normal lung markings can be seen, becoming denser at the lung base. The contour of the left hemidiaphragm is still lost.

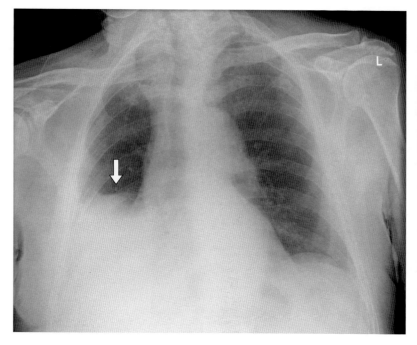

Fig. 20.4 Subpulmonic effusion – different patient. This is an even more difficult appearance of an effusion– the fluid is all below the hemidiaphragm in the inferior pleural space – a subpulmonic effusion.

This has the appearance of a raised hemidiaphragm (arrow), with no lung markings below it (usually lung markings can be seen here). The contour of the apparently raised hemidiaphragm may be indistinct.

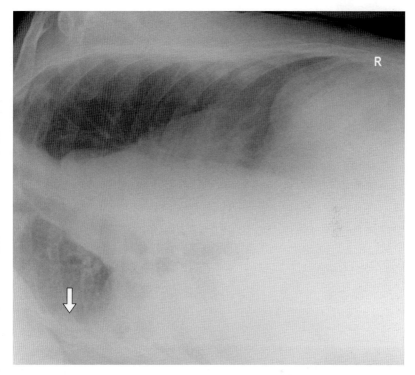

Fig. 20.5 Confirmation of the presence of a subpulmonic effusion may be confirmed with a lateral decubitus film with the patient lying on the side of the proposed effusion. This causes the fluid to collect dependently (arrow). This is the same patient as Fig. 20.4.

Important management points and further investigations

Immediate management

Place the patient on oxygen if there is respiratory compromise.

This condition does not usually require immediate action, although further investigation and treatment may be required.

Further management considerations

A chest drain may need to be placed (see Chapter 5) if the effusion is symptomatic.

Pleural fluid can be aspirated (or collected when a drain is inserted) and sent to the laboratory for culture and biochemical analysis as well as cytology.

Further imaging

Ultrasound may be considered to confirm the presence of an effusion and to mark a suitable position for a drain. Most drains are placed under US guidance.

CT may be helpful to find a cause (such as malignancy).

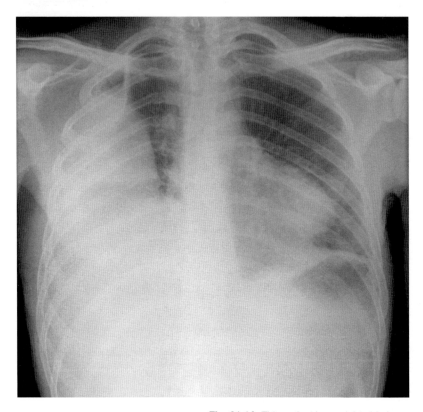

Fig. 21.1A This patient has a right-sided empyema, with some air within it superiorly.

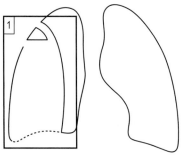

Background

Empyema refers to an infected pleural space collection, and as such most commonly accompanies pneumonia (see Chapter 8). The condition carries a high mortality rate and appropriate management is by drainage of the empyema.

Clinical features

Signs and symptoms are those of pneumonia with an effusion. The patient is usually unwell.

Differential diagnosis

- Uncomplicated pleural effusion (Chapter 20)
- Lung abscess can be difficult to differentiate (Chapter 10).

Radiological features

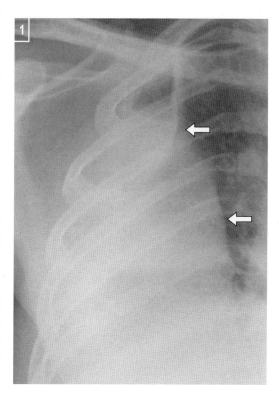

Fig. 21.1B This patient has a fluid collection in the pleural space. The classic appearance of an empyema is of a lobulated pleural space collection, with convex contours (arrows).

The patient also has air within the pleural space collection superiorly from previous attempted aspiration in this case.

Important management points and further investigations

Immediate management

Empyemas need to be drained. Liaise with your senior. The patient may require further imaging.

Accepted methods of treatment include insertion of a large-bore drain, insertion of a small drain and urokinase through the drain into the pleural space, or video-assisted thoracoscopy (VATS).

Further imaging

Ultrasound can help to determine whether a collection is echogenic and contains debris and whether there are loculations, which can occur in chronic empyemas.

CT is the gold standard for diagnosis and can be used to differentiate between lung abscess and empyema.

22 Pericardial effusion

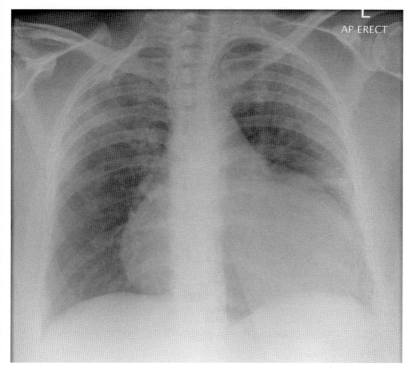

Fig. 22.1 This radiograph demonstrates a water-bottle-shaped heart in a young patient who was subsequently shown to have a pericardial effusion at echocardiography.

Background

Pericardial effusion is defined as abnormal fluid in the pericardial space.

There are several causes including trauma, inflammation, malignancy and autoimmune conditions. It can also accompany pericarditis.

This is an important condition because it may lead to cardiac tamponade, as the build-up of fluid restricts normal cardiac motion.

Clinical features

Symptoms

These are non-specific and include shortness of breath, chest discomfort and palpitations.

Signs

Look for the signs of cardiac tamponade (Beck's triad): hypotension, muffled heart sounds and raised JVP.

A pericardial rub may be heard if the patient has pericarditis.

Radiological features

Remember that a CXR is not the best way to diagnose this condition. However, in a patient with non-specific signs and symptoms, noticing the classic signs and arranging further imaging may benefit your patient.

The classic CXR appearance is that of a water-bottle-shaped heart but this is not very specific. Any cause of cardiomegaly can look similar. But be aware of this diagnosis in a young patient with cardiomegaly as the patient can quickly become compromised.

The message is simple – if there is a big heart on the CXR think of this diagnosis.

A pleural effusion frequently accompanies this finding.

The heart will have a very sharply demarcated outline because the fluid masks the blurring caused by cardiac motion. Differential diagnosis includes dilated cardiomyopathy with generalized chamber enlargement and poor contractility. Look for evidence of left atrial enlargement (splaying of the tracheal bifurcation and elevation of the left main bronchus), which will be absent in pericardial effusion but may be present in dilated cardiomyopathy.

An echocardiogram can be arranged to confirm the diagnosis.

Important management points and further investigations

Immediate management

Principles are as follows:

- Ensure the patient is stable. If there are any signs of cardiovascular compromise involve a senior immediately.
- Perform an ECG to look for evidence of pericarditis – saddle-shaped ST elevation, which may help confirm the diagnosis.
- Arrange prompt definitive imaging.
- Seek and treat the underlying cause, which may be evident from the past medical history.

Further management considerations

- Consider requesting a cardiology opinion.
- Non-steroidal anti-inflammatory drugs (NSAIDs) may be helpful.
- Pericardiocentesis may be considered.

Further imaging

- Echocardiography may be considered as a first line.
- CT and MRI are also sensitive.

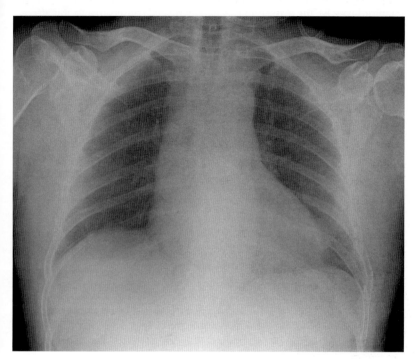

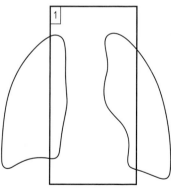

Fig. 23.1A This radiograph demonstrates widening of the mediastinum caused by a thoracic aortic dissection.

Background

This is an important condition with a high mortality rate. Untreated mortality is 50% in the first 24 hours.

There are several causes including Marfan syndrome, Ehlers–Danlos syndrome and iatrogenic trauma.

Classification and further management depends on which parts of the aorta are affected. If the dissection commences distal to the left subclavian artery (Stanford type B), the dissection is generally treated conservatively; if it affects the ascending aortic arch (Stanford type A), operative treatment is indicated.

As these patients generally present with chest pain they can be mistakenly treated for acute coronary syndrome. A high clinical and radiological index of suspicion is required for accurate diagnosis.

Clinical features

Aortic dissection generally affects people between 40 and 70 years of age. There is a male to female ratio of 3 to 1.

Signs and symptoms

There is sudden-onset tearing chest pain radiating to the back, with the pain being worst at onset. The pain may also be interscapular.

Signs and symptoms may also reflect involvement of branches of the aorta, e.g. Horner's syndrome (carotid), neurology (carotid), secondary myocardial infarct (coronary).

Check the blood pressure in each arm to look for a difference between the sides.

Differential diagnosis

Any cause of chest pain is a differential. Acute coronary syndromes are common and often do not present classically.

Thoracic aortic aneurysms and traumatic aortic rupture can look similar on the CXR, manifesting as a widened mediastinum.

Radiological features

The CXR is abnormal in 80% of patients with dissection.

Do not rely on the CXR – signs are subtle and the diagnosis should be based on clinical findings as well as imaging.

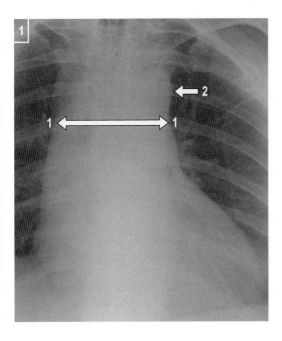

Fig. 23.1B The widened mediastinum is the classic finding in patients with thoracic aortic dissection. However, remember that such patients will often have undergone an AP film, which makes assessment of the mediastinum difficult owing to magnification.

A diameter of over 8 cm is concerning (arrow 1). Look at the width of the mediastinum compared to the cardiac silhouette to get an idea if it is too large. The aortic knuckle may also be indistinct or lost (arrow 2).

Other signs to look for include an area of increased density at the left apex – a pleural cap, deviation of the trachea to the left and depression of the left main bronchus.

Important management points and further investigations

Immediate management

- Patients require immediate resuscitation with oxygen, and intravenous access/intravenous fluids.
- Inform your senior.
- A cardiothoracic surgical opinion is advised.

Further management considerations

The patient will require definitive imaging for diagnosis.

Beta-blockers can be considered, to reduce the blood pressure and thus the likelihood of propagation.

Further imaging

CT aortography will demonstrate the dissection if present, and determine what type it is and what further management is indicated, as well as demonstrating complications such as haemothorax and cardiac tamponade.

If the patient is unstable a doctor should accompany the patient to the CT unit.

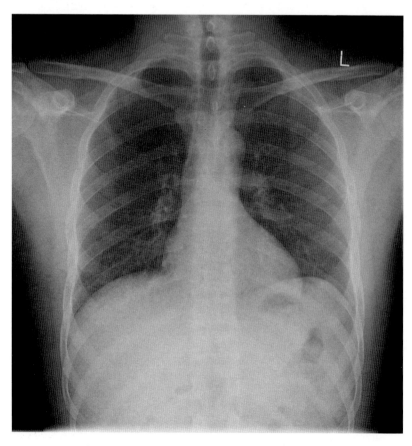

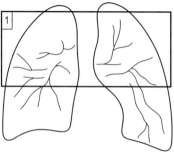

Fig. 24.1A This radiograph demonstrates a very subtle area of oligaemia in the right upper zone, with a decreased vessel count. The subsequent CT pulmonary angiogram demonstrated a right-sided pulmonary embolus.

Background

Pulmonary embolism (PE) is a serious condition and a leading cause of mortality. It is important for all on-call doctors to be familiar with this condition, as it can occur in any inpatient. It is a common postoperative complication and a common reason for admission to hospital.

Algorithms for clinical assessment of PE and the role of simple tests and imaging are often poorly understood.

Clinical features

Clinical signs and symptoms are non-specific and a high index of suspicion for this condition is necessary.

Remember to seek risk factors: malignancy, immobility, coagulopathies, recent surgery (this list is not exhaustive).

Symptoms

Symptoms include dyspnoea, pleuritic chest pain and haemoptysis; their onset is usually sudden.

Signs

Chest wall tenderness may occur. The patient may also have tachypnoea, tachycardia and hypoxia. Massive PE may be associated with hypotension and raised JVP.

Differential diagnosis

The following conditions should be excluded – some can be diagnosed using simple tests before asking for a CT pulmonary angiogram:

- myocardial infarction/acute coronary syndrome – consider ECG and troponins
- pneumothorax – CXR to rule out (see Chapter 18).
- pneumonia – history may be different (productive cough and high fever), and CXR (although consolidation may look like infarction) (see Chapter 8)
- aortic dissection – widened mediastinum on CXR, different history (see Chapter 23)
- pericarditis – central pain of insidious onset, saddle-shaped ST segments on ECG
- acute asthma – diagnosis may be known, there is an expiratory wheeze, and the condition improves with use of a nebulizer (although wheeze can occur in PE)
- rib fractures – may be seen on the CXR and there should be a preceding history of trauma.

There are many more differentials.

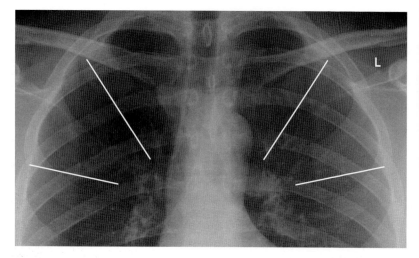

Fig. 24.1B In this patient the area between the lines is more radiolucent and contains fewer vessels on the right. This is very subtle and is the most common CXR abnormality (if the CXR is abnormal). Differential diagnosis of this appearance includes an area of emphysema or bullous change in the lung (see Chapters 14 and 18).

Radiological features

A CXR should be performed urgently in all patients with suspected PE. There are two reasons for this:

1. You may diagnose an alternative pathology, such as pneumothorax, pneumonia or rib fractures.
2. The first-line complex imaging modality is a ventilation/perfusion (V/Q) scan, or increasingly, CT pulmonary angiogram (CTPA). A normal chest x-ray is required to interpret the V/Q scan. Parenchymal CXR abnormalities may cause defects on the V/Q scan which may render this test indeterminate. *Most CXRs in patients with pulmonary emboli are normal.*

There may be subtle signs of a PE on a plain radiograph, but these are generally non-specific.

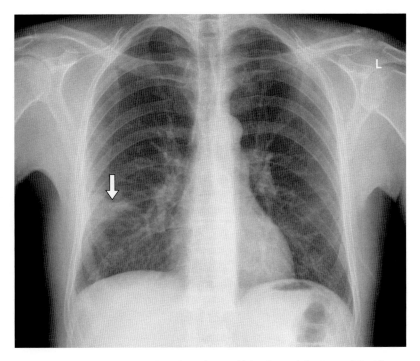

Fig. 24.2 This patient has a wedge-shaped area of infarction pointing toward the hilum. This is called Hampton's hump (arrow). (With thanks to Dr Emma Lawrence for providing this radiograph.)

Other signs

There may be a wedge-shaped area of oligaemia, and an adjacent area of hyperaemia (Westermark's sign).

The pulmonary artery is sometimes distended in patients with pulmonary embolism.

Important management points and further investigations

Immediate management

Prompt management is the key. If you suspect a massive PE, consider urgent definitive imaging after having performed basic resuscitative manoeuvres (oxygen, fluids).

If the diagnosis is suspected, empirical treatment with treatment-dose low molecular weight heparin should be instigated. Remember that aortic dissection should be excluded before commencing such therapy (see Chapter 23).

Perform an ECG. Abnormalities such as sinus tachycardia, atrial fibrillation, right axis deviation, right bundle branch block and a right strain pattern are suggestive. The 'classic' S1Q3T3 pattern is rare. You may also diagnose myocardial infarction/ischaemia.

Arterial blood gas analysis will confirm hypoxia. This is easier to interpret with the patient off oxygen therapy temporarily but if the patient is significantly hypoxic do not interrupt oxygen therapy.

The d-dimer is a poorly understood test and should not be used in isolation to make clinical decisions. It has a good negative predictive value – so if the d-dimer is normal, the patient is unlikely to have a PE. However, if the d-dimer is raised, the positive predictive value is poor. A raised d-dimer is non-specific and can be raised in a variety of conditions, such as postoperative patients, malignancy and infection which are all common. A positive d-dimer is not necessarily indicative of a PE, although there is evidence that a very high d-dimer is suggestive.

Further imaging

V/Q scanning is considered the first-line complex imaging modality although a normal chest radiograph is a prerequisite.

The result will come back as high, intermediate or low probability, or normal, and this should be interpreted in the context of the clinical probability.

'High probability' normally leads to treatment (85% chance of a PE), intermediate probability requires another test (usually a CTPA). Low probability indicates an approximately 9% chance of a PE and virtually excludes a PE if the clinical probability is low.

CTPA is the gold standard but requires a large volume of intravenous contrast. CTPA can also be inconclusive. The pulmonary vessels are opacified using CTPA and clots can be visualized. CTPA is used as a first line if the CXR is abnormal.

Further reading

Sensitivity and specificity of definitive tests has been assessed in the PIOPED (Prospective Investigation of Pulmonary Embolism Diagnosis) trial. PIOPED II is of particular interest as it examines CTPA and V/Q scintigraphy.

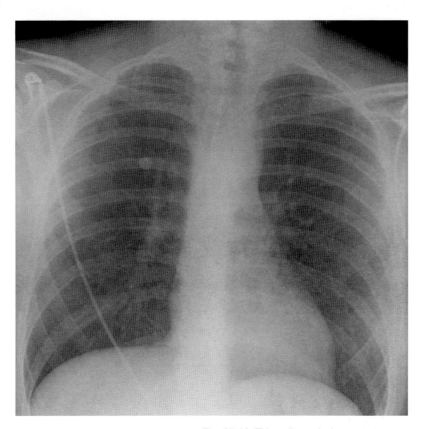

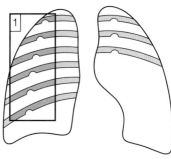

Fig. 25.1A This radiograph demonstrates inferior rib notching bilaterally. The diagnosis is coarctation of the aorta.

Background

Coarctation of the aorta does not usually present as an emergency but if you spot the abnormality it might make a big difference to the patient.

The pathology is narrowing of the aorta, usually just distal to the origin of the left subclavian artery. This in turn causes increased afterload on the heart and heart failure (See Ch. 26). These patients also present with hypertension.

It may present with cardiac failure in childhood. In infants, increased left ventricular strain and left to right shunting of blood through a patent ductus arteriosus, which lies proximal to the coarctation, can lead to biventricular high output cardiac failure.

Coarctation may present with hypertension later in life and is a diagnosis that is difficult to make and is often missed.

It is also often associated with heart defects.

Clinical features

In infants there is failure to thrive and feed progressing to cardiac failure. It may present acutely. Patients can present in shock.

It can also present later with hypertension, which is often discovered incidentally.

Look for poor distal pulses and radiofemoral delay. There may be a discrepancy in blood pressure measurements between the arms. There may also be clinical evidence of associated congenital heart disease.

Radiological features

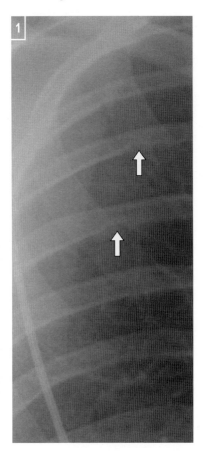

Fig. 25.1B The classic finding is notching of the inferior ribs in the region of the internal thoracic arteries (arrows). These have a raised pressure due to the coarctation causing pressure erosions of the ribs. The aortic knuckle may also be abnormal and resemble a figure 3 (not seen in this example). The inferior aspects of the ribs are an important review area.

This appearance is usually seen in patients presenting with hypertension where pressure erosion of the ribs has had time to develop (not usually before the age of 10 years).

Other conditions can cause rib notching without coarctation, such as neurofibromatosis, where the notching is due to pressure from multiple tumours of the intercostal nerves.

Important management points and further investigations

Immediate management

Patients with coarctation of the aorta may eventually require surgical correction so this finding is important. However, they may not be acutely ill at presentation.

Further management considerations

If the diagnosis is confirmed, a cardiothoracic opinion is advised.

Further imaging

Cardiac MRI or CT scanning will help to confirm the diagnosis.

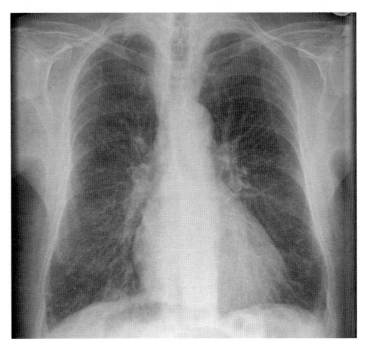

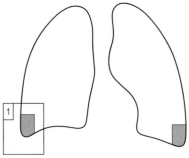

Fig. 26.1A Pulmonary oedema due to heart failure. Mild.

Background

The commonest causes of pulmonary oedema encountered by the on-call doctor are cardiac failure and iatrogenic fluid overload. The latter should be clear within its clinical context. Cardiogenic pulmonary oedema coexists with cardiac enlargement. See the section on PA versus AP projection, Chapter 6, page 37.

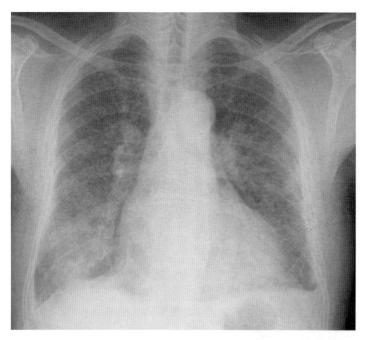

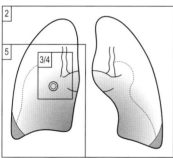

Fig. 26.1B Pulmonary oedema due to heart failure. Moderate.

Pulmonary oedema can develop quickly (e.g. associated with myocardial infarct, renal failure/artery stenosis) or more slowly (gradual fluid overload due to cardiac failure).

Clinical features

Symptoms

Symptoms include dyspnoea, orthopnoea, paroxysmal nocturnal dyspnoea and peripheral oedema.

The clinical context is important: Is the patient on fluids following surgery? Is there a known history of cardiac or renal failure, or of fever or drowning?

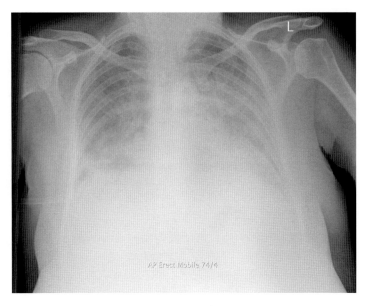

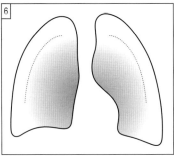

Fig. 26.1C Pulmonary oedema due to heart failure. Severe.

Signs

The main signs are fine basal crackles, raised JVP, added heart sounds, murmurs (cause or effect), displaced apex beat and peripheral oedema.

These patients can present to almost any on-call doctor – medical admission or wards, postoperative patients given too much fluid, and the ED.

Differential diagnosis

Any cause of fluid in the alveoli can give the appearance of 'airspace shadowing' on the CXR. This causes areas of soft tissue density (grey-white) on the background air density (black).

The lung changes seen in cardiac failure are generally bilateral and symmetrical in distribution, but may be asymmetrical with right-sided changes predominating. There are also several other radiological clues described below.

Other types of fluid in the alveoli can cause unilateral or bilateral but often asymmetric airspace shadowing, for example pus in pneumonia (Chapter 8) blood in contusion and bronchioloalveolar carcinoma.

It is important to correlate these findings with the patient's clinical features in order to make the correct diagnosis.

Remember as well that pneumonia and heart failure may coexist and serial CXRs may be necessary for diagnosis. Pulmonary oedema is more fleeting than consolidation radiographically and with treatment will resolve quickly. Even with treatment, the radiographic changes of pneumonia will persist for longer.

Radiological features

There are several patterns of cardiac failure. We have divided these into early (mild), moderate and late (severe) but in reality all of the signs should be sought as they can all coexist.

Look at old films if available and consider repeat radiography after diuretic treatment as heart failure is generally a more fleeting process than pneumonia, which is its main differential.

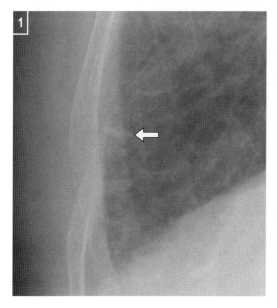

Fig. 26.2A Mild pulmonary oedema. This patient has septal lines or Kerley B lines. These represent fluid in the interlobular septa and are a very early sign of fluid overload. They are normally seen at the costophrenic angle but can be seen subpleurally further up the chest (arrow). Kerley B lines can also be seen in interstitial processes such as fibrosis but in the correct clinical setting (clinical features as above, enlarged heart) their aetiology should be clear. Resolution after treatment is an added clue. This is the only sign of heart failure in the lungs in this patient.

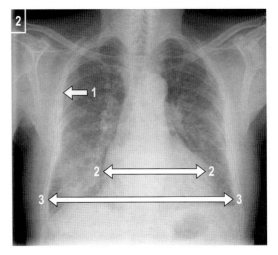

Fig. 26.2B Moderate pulmonary oedema. The film has been taken with a PA projection as the scapulae are excluded and do not overlap the thorax (arrow 1). The ratio of the cardiac diameter (arrow 2) and the thoracic diameter (arrow 3) is in excess of 0.5 on this PA film so the heart is genuinely enlarged.

Fig. 26.1A also demonstrates cardiac enlargement but is more difficult to assess as the film has been taken AP.

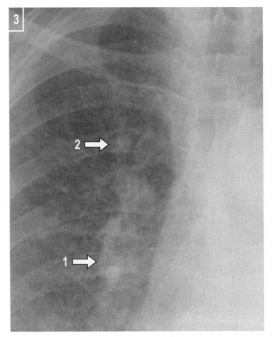

Fig. 26.2C Moderate pulmonary oedema. The hila can be enlarged due to central venous congestion. This is observed bilaterally (arrow 1).

Also seen in most stages of heart failure is the phenomenon of upper lobe diversion. In fluid overload the upper lobe vessels are larger than the lower lobe ones and this is also due to venous congestion (arrow 2).

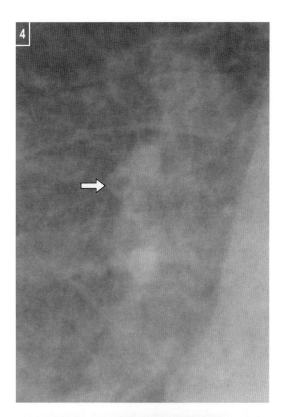

Fig. 26.2D Moderate pulmonary oedema. Peribronchial cuffing is seen in early and moderate heart failure. It is another example of the silhouette sign (see p. 4).

In normal chest x-rays the bronchi are thin-walled and not particularly conspicuous, contain air, and are superimposed against the air containing alveoli. In cardiac failure the alveoli are filled with water. This collects around the bronchus so the bronchi going toward or away from the viewer are now seen end-on as a ring shadow – with a 'cuff' of fluid (arrow).

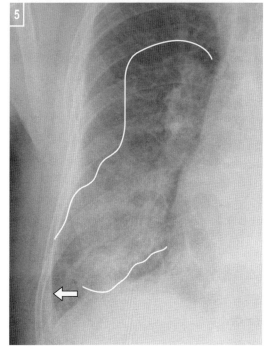

Fig. 26.2E Moderate pulmonary oedema. An example of moderate airspace shadowing. In heart failure the shadowing or whiteness is seen adjacent to the hila and at the lung bases (outlined). Airspace shadowing in heart failure is generally symmetrical as outlined. However, it can be unilateral if the patient has been lying on one side. Look for all the other clues.

Patients with heart failure develop pleural effusions which whilst usually bilateral can also be quite asymmetrical (arrow), usually larger on the left (see also Chapter 20).

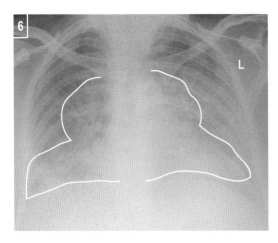

Fig. 26.2F Severe pulmonary oedema. Advanced cardiac failure has a perihilar and/or basal distribution as illustrated.

It can be purely perihilar where it is described as 'bat wing' shadowing.

Important management points and further investigations

Immediate management

Pulmonary oedema is one of the commonest diagnostic and management scenarios encountered by the on-call junior doctor. Do not hesitate to involve your senior if you are unsure; the radiologist may also be able to help with the diagnosis.

The immediate treatment of cardiogenic pulmonary oedema is oxygen and diuretics and/or vasodilators.

With appropriate treatment, the clinical and radiological features of pulmonary oedema resolve quickly.

Further imaging

Plain films are usually all that is necessary for diagnosis. Follow-up radiography can be useful both for confirming the diagnosis and for assessing response to treatment.

Echocardiography will help quantify and confirm the presence of cardiac dysfunction.

Further reading

Gluecker T, Capasso P, Schnyder P, et al. Clinical and radiologic features of pulmonary edema. Radiographics 1999;19:1507–31.

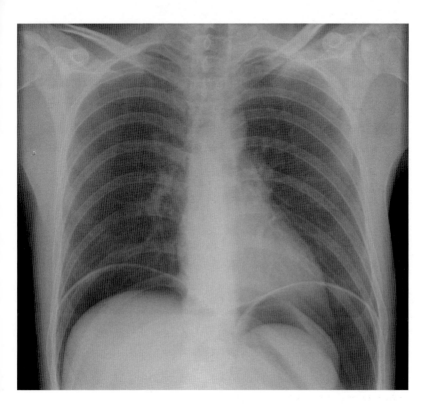

Fig. 27.1A Pneumoperitoneum on an
erect chest X-ray.

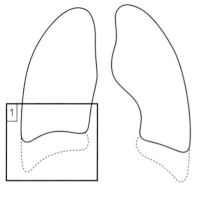

Background

The erect chest x-ray is the most important plain film for diagnosis of perforated abdominal viscus.

The patient needs to be erect for 5 minutes before a chest radiograph is taken. It does not matter if the radiograph is AP or PA. If there is a perforated viscus, air will rise and collect beneath one or both hemidiaphragms.

This technique is about 80% sensitive for perforation. Lateral films are reportedly more sensitive for detection of pneumoperitoneum [1] but rarely performed in practice.

The commonest causes of air under the diaphragm are perforated peptic ulcer (large volume of air), perforated diverticular disease (smaller amount of air) and perforation of obstructed bowel (small or large bowel).

The presence of pneumoperitoneum usually mandates an exploratory laparotomy. However, remember that there are causes of air under the diaphragm for which an operation is not necessary. These include recent laparotomy/laparoscopy, pneumatosis coli, peritoneal dialysis (look for a peritoneal dialysis tube and appropriate history), and entry through the female genital tract (again the history will determine this).

Clinical features

Symptoms

There is abdominal pain, of sudden onset. Because the pain of peritonitis irritates the parietal peritoneum, the patient will prefer to lie still and will experience pain on movement.

Pain may be referred to the shoulder tip due to diaphragmatic irritation.

Signs

- Signs of peritonism (guarding, rebound, rigid abdomen, silent abdomen).
- Shock. Beware the patient on steroids, who may have few signs or symptoms.

Radiological features

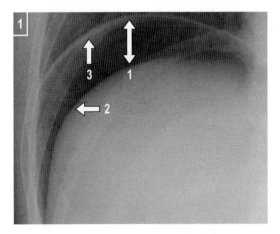

Fig. 27.1B Air collects under the hemidiaphragm (arrow 1). The upper border of the liver is outlined by free air superiorly (arrow 2). The thin diaphragmatic outline is seen, outlined by air underneath it (free air) and air above it in the lung (arrow 3).

The continuous diaphragm sign may be seen in pneumoperitoneum as well as pneumopericardium as free intraperitoneal air outlines the undersurface of the central diaphragm (see p. 104).

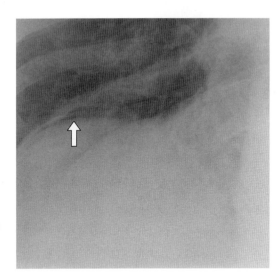

Fig. 27.2 In this different patient there is a small amount of free air under the right hemidiaphragm. Look carefully for small amounts of air (arrow).

There are a number of mimics of free subdiaphragmatic air (see over leaf).

Mimics of perforation and pitfalls
Normal fundal bubble

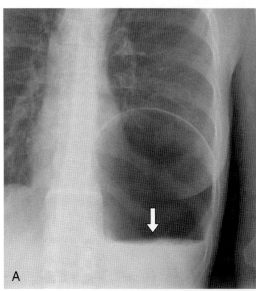

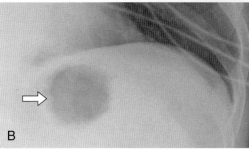

Fig. 27.3A and B Looking under the right hemidiaphragm for free air is often easiest as the normal fundal bubble can cause confusion. The gastric fundus normally contains a bubble of air.

This air will, however, have the characteristics of air in the fundus of the stomach. Its shape will be limited by the shape of the stomach (**B**) so it will not be crescentic as seen with the perforation (see Fig. 27.1A).

There may also be an air–fluid level (arrow, **A**) in the fundus of the stomach, and food debris may even be seen. Gastric rugae can sometimes also be seen outlined by air (arrow, **B**).

A fundal bubble and free air can coexist – suspect a perforation when two collections of air are seen under the left hemidiaphragm, one not within the stomach.

Chilaiditi sign

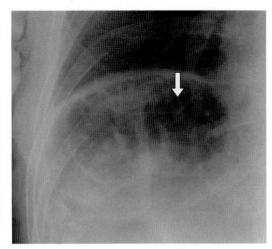

Fig. 27.4 Free air under the right hemidiaphragm is not always straightforward though.

Colon between the upper liver and diaphragm can simulate a perforation. However, the normal anatomical features of colon can be seen in the form of haustrae (arrow), which differentiate colon from free air.

Basal atelectasis

This can lead to confusion as a horizontal band of atelectasis at the lung base can simulate diaphragm, and the lung between the atelectasis and actual diaphragm can look like free air.

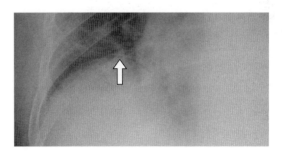

Fig. 27.5 A very thin crescent of lung base between what is obviously atelectasis and the hemidiaphragm simulates the crescent seen in this patient (arrow).

Lateral decubitus films may assist in differentiating basal atelectasis and pneumoperitoneum (see Chapters 20 and 45).

Important management points and further investigations

Immediate management

Pneumoperitoneum is an emergency and if suspected your senior needs to be involved.

Prompt referral to the general surgeon is important. These patients generally require a laparotomy and must be adequately resuscitated before theatre.

Further management considerations

An AXR may be of value in diagnosis. It may diagnose an obstruction responsible for the free air, and signs of perforation may be seen on an AXR (see Chapter 45). An AXR and erect CXR are usually both done if perforation is suspected.

Obtain the help of your senior or a radiologist to make the radiological diagnosis as it may not be straightforward.

Further imaging

CT may be helpful in equivocal cases of perforation or to find a cause, particularly if the patient is obstructed. If there is an unequivocal pneumoperitoneum on plain films, further imaging should not delay prompt laparotomy.

CT is more sensitive than CXR or AXR for detection of pneumoperitoneum [2] so if radiographs are negative and clinical suspicion is strong, CT should be considered. Remember first to exclude other causes of peritonitis, such as pancreatitis.

Discuss further imaging on a case-by-case basis with your senior and radiologist.

References

[1] Woodring JH, Heiser MJ. Detection of pneumoperitoneum on chest radiographs: comparison of upright and lateral chest radiographs. AJR Am J Roentgenol 1995;165:45–7.
[2] Stapakis JC, Thickman D. Diagnosis of pneumoperitoneum: abdominal CT versus upright chest film. J Comput Assist Tomogr 1992;16(5):713–6.

Abdominal x-rays

28 System for interpretation of the AXR

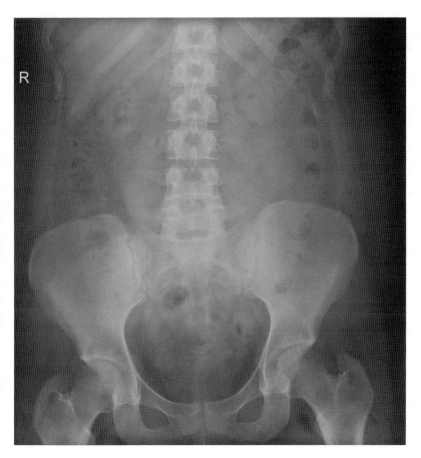

Fig. 28.1 A normal AXR.

This chapter aims to provide the reader with a checklist of structures to look at when interpreting an AXR.

Technical factors

The abdomen is almost exclusively soft tissue with air in the GI tract. Radiographic exposure factors are less critical than for the CXR.

It is important to ensure that the whole abdomen is imaged, including the hernial orifices (the radiograph should include the whole bony pelvis).

Also bear in mind that detail on the AXR in obese patients may be suboptimal.

Structures can be subtle in the abdomen as all organs are of soft tissue density and can only be seen because of subtle differences in thickness and density. Some organs are surrounded by fat, which can help.

Start by assessing any lines or tubes – these may include a PEG tube, or abdominal drains, catheters etc.

Organs that can be seen

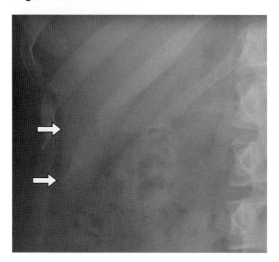

Fig. 28.2 The liver edge is subtle but can be seen (arrows). Look for liver enlargement.

Look in the region of the liver for abnormal gas in the biliary tree (see Chapter 31) or portal venous gas (see Chapter 37), which can be a poor prognostic sign in various conditions.

Look for gallstones in the region of the gallbladder.

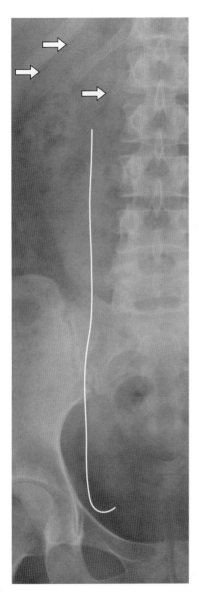

Fig. 28.3 The renal outline can also be seen, usually just lateral to the upper psoas shadow. It can be seen because it is surrounded by fat in the perinephric space (arrows). The renal outline is important for a number of reasons. Kidney stones may be seen projected over the kidney. The kidney may also be enlarged, as in polycystic kidney disease. Look for gas in emphysematous pyelonephritis (Chapter 40).

Knowledge of the course of the ureter is also important as a stone can be found at any point along its length. The ureter emerges from the medial aspect of the kidney and descends into the pelvis at the level of the tips of the transverse processes of the lumbar vertebrae. The ureter then crosses the pelvic brim and turns inward to enter the bladder at the level of the ischial spine. Use these landmarks to help you. The approximate course of the ureter is drawn in.

Ultrasound is the best initial modality for investigating renal disease.

The splenic outline may also be seen in the left upper quadrant, particularly if enlarged.

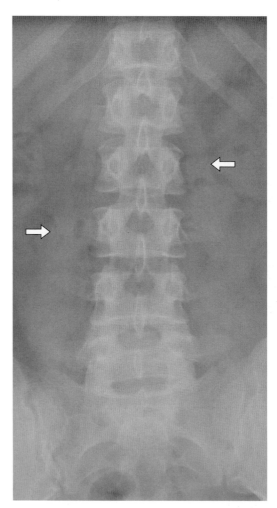

Fig. 28.4 Always look in the midline for the outline of a calcified aorta.

An aneurysm may be the cause of the patient's pain and this diagnosis may be quickly lethal. See Chapter 42.

The psoas shadows can also be seen. This can be a useful sign as their obliteration can indicate pathology in the retroperitoneum such as blood (arrows), although loss of psoas outline is not a particularly sensitive or specific sign.

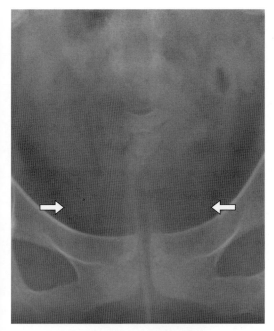

Fig. 28.5 The bladder may also be seen. In this case it is not very full but it may be seen as a rounded viscus in the pelvis (arrows). Stones can sometimes be seen in the bladder.

Look for mural gas in emphysematous cystitis – see Chapter 39.

A soft tissue density seen above the bladder in a female patient may represent the uterus.

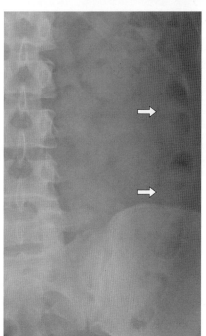

Fig. 28.6 Look at the bowel gas pattern.

The colon is peripheral, larger and more fixed in position than the small bowel (arrows). It may contain faeces, which are mottled in density.

Look for large bowel obstruction (Chapter 32) and signs of inflammatory bowel disease (Chapter 35) as well as volvulus (Chapters 33 and 34).

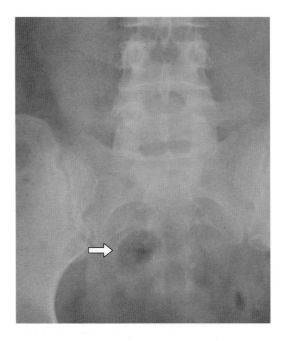

Fig. 28.7 Normal small bowel has locules of air within it. Small bowel is variable in position as it is on a mesentery (arrow). Look for signs of small bowel obstruction (Chapter 30).

A paucity of bowel gas can also be a bad sign – it may represent late obstruction, where the bowel loops fill with fluid.

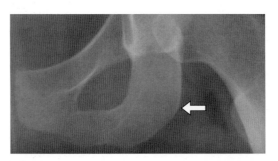

Fig. 28.8 Check the hernial orifices for hernias – seen as locules of air in loops of bowel in this region (arrow) (see Chapter 30).

Check the bones for metastases and fractures.

Look for abnormal air, which might indicate a perforation (see Chapter 45). If this is suspected the AXR is usually performed with an accompanying erect CXR.

29 Gastric outlet obstruction

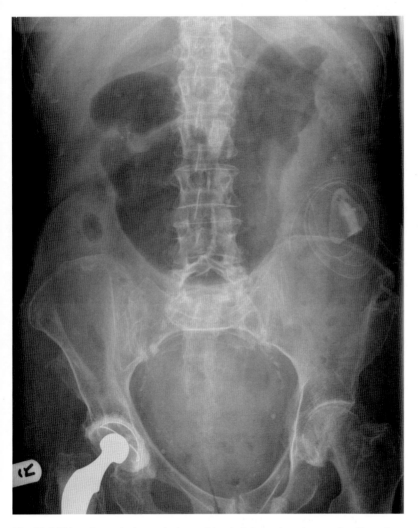

Fig. 29.1 This radiograph demonstrates a distended stomach and a paucity of bowel gas elsewhere. This patient has gastric outlet obstruction (strictly speaking in this case the obstruction is probably just distal to the stomach as gas is seen in the duodenal cap). Note the jejunostomy and right total hip replacement.

Gastric outlet obstruction is defined as any process that impedes emptying of the stomach. Its causes are similar to those of intestinal obstruction – functional and mechanical.

Diabetic gastroparesis and ileus/pseudo-obstruction are functional causes of obstruction.

Mechanical causes can be divided into benign and malignant. The commonest benign cause is peptic ulcer disease leading to scarring and pyloric stenosis. Pancreatic pseudocysts can also cause the same appearances. Malignant causes include pancreatic and gastric tumours as well as metastases.

Clinical features

Symptoms

Patients present with non-bilious vomiting, often shortly after ingestion of a meal, with relatively undigested food in the vomitus. Weight loss may be a feature. Patients may aspirate.

Symptomatology may point to the underlying cause.

Signs

A succussion splash may be evident. A mass may also be evident, and the patient may be dehydrated.

Differential diagnosis

Causes are described above.

Intestinal obstruction may present in a similar fashion and is commoner but is usually associated with bilious or faeculent vomiting.

Radiological features

The stomach may be filled with air (as above) or food debris.

Do not confuse the stomach with the transverse colon. As can be seen on the radiograph, its shape is distinctive.

Important management points and further investigations

Immediate management

Decompression with a nasogastric tube is advised. Replace fluids. Correct metabolic alkalosis and electrolyte disturbance.

Further management considerations

Further diagnosis may be made with endoscopy or an upper GI contrast study/CT.

Involve a surgeon with management.

Further imaging

Upper GI contrast study or CT may be helpful. Upper GI endoscopy may also be considered.

30 Small bowel obstruction

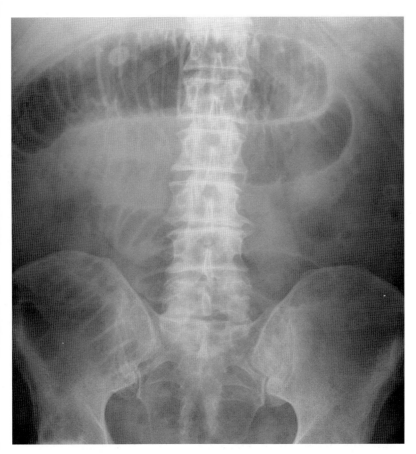

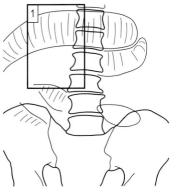

Fig. 30.1A The radiograph shows several abnormally dilated small bowel loops in small bowel obstruction.

Background

Small bowel obstruction is a very common emergency presentation and as plain films are still the first-line modality for diagnosis, accurate interpretation is important to enable prompt, accurate management of these patients.

Causes may be mechanical or functional (due to a paralysis of the bowel wall). The commonest two causes of mechanical obstruction are adhesions and hernias. Tumours (of the small bowel or caecum, or metastatic) are also a common cause. The finding of small bowel obstruction should prompt the assessing physician to elicit a history of malignancy or previous surgery (adhesions) and examine the groins (for hernias).

Functional obstruction most commonly follows abdominal surgery, which should be clear clinically. Pseudo-obstruction is a condition that has several underlying causes such as electrolyte disturbances and fractures. It is difficult to differentiate this from mechanical obstruction on radiological grounds alone.

Be aware of the complication of perforation – longstanding small bowel obstruction leads to bowel ischaemia and necrosis which may initially manifest as pneumatosis intestinalis (see Chapter 37). Do not forget to request an erect CXR in patients with suspected obstruction and look for the signs of perforation (see Chapters 27 and 45).

Clinical features

Symptoms

The main symptoms are colicky central abdominal pain, vomiting, absolute constipation and abdominal distension.

Signs

Signs include a distended tympanic abdomen and increased, tinkling bowel sounds on auscultation, as distinct from ileus or functional obstruction where bowel sounds are absent. Look for scars indicating previous surgery and hernias.

Peritonism may suggest perforation, which may complicate obstruction.

In very late presentation small bowel obstruction, bowel sounds may be decreased or absent.

Differential diagnosis

Large bowel obstruction is a radiological and clinical differential (see Chapter 32).

Radiological features

Remember the order of events in small bowel obstruction as this will explain the radiological features of small bowel obstruction, which vary with time.

Imagine the bowel as a tube. If it becomes obstructed, there is firstly a build-up of air behind the obstruction and the bowel gradually increases in calibre. A diameter of over 2.5 cm is considered dilated. Therefore, a length of gas-filled dilated bowel is abnormal (gas in the small bowel is usually in small pockets).

Eventually the bowel proximal to the obstruction becomes fluid-filled and much harder to see (remembering from silhouette signs that differences in density are required to see things clearly on radiographs, see p. 3–4). However, with a high index of suspicion and a keen eye, dilated fluid-filled bowel loops can sometimes be seen.

It should be remembered that for this reason an apparently normal AXR does not exclude small bowel obstruction and in this scenario (plain films are only about 50–60% sensitive [1] – low-grade obstructions and fluid-filled bowel loops being the most difficult scenarios), if the diagnosis is suspected clinically, CT is more sensitive.

Radiography can demonstrate the presence of small bowel obstruction but will not generally demonstrate the cause. Two exceptions include gallstone ileus (see Chapter 31), where the diagnosis is a radiological one, and hernias (always look in the hernial orifices both on the plain film and the patient).

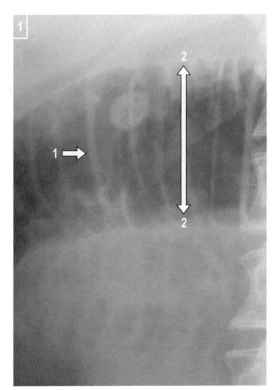

Fig. 30.1B The ability to differentiate between dilated small and large bowel is important for interpretation. Small bowel is generally central, and the small bowel contains valvulae conniventes which traverse the entire diameter of the bowel (arrow 1). In colonic loops the mucosal folds are called haustrae and do not traverse the bowel lumen completely.

A diameter of over 2.5 cm suggests obstruction (arrow 2).

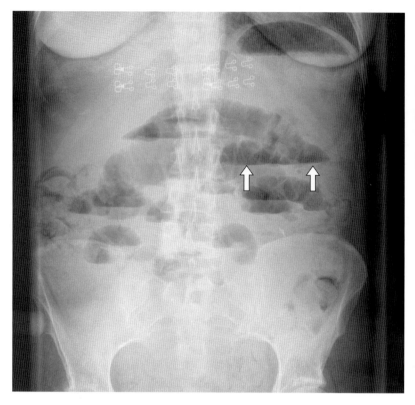

Fig. 30.2 Erect abdominal x-ray, from a different patient. If there is diagnostic doubt, an erect film may help. Remember that in obstruction the loops proximal to the obstruction fill first with air, then with fluid, so sitting the patient upright will enable the air–fluid levels (arrows) to be seen as the air rises to the top and the fluid settles to the bottom. This cannot be seen in the standard supine film.

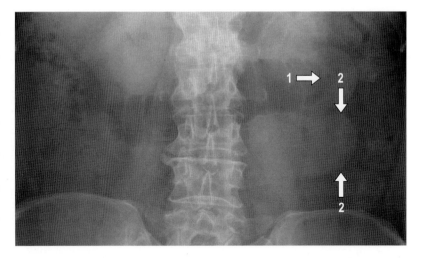

Fig. 30.3 This patient has more advanced small bowel obstruction. The gas-filled loop in the upper abdomen shows the gaseous distension of early obstruction and one can see it is partially fluid filled on this supine film (arrow 1). The loop below it is completely fluid filled (arrows 2) and as such it is more difficult to see. In advanced obstruction the abdomen may appear 'gasless'.

When the bowel loop is almost filled with fluid and has only a little gas within it, small bubbles of gas may be seen 'trapped' under successive valvulae conniventes. This appearance is called the 'string of pearls' sign. It is seen relatively uncommonly on plain films.

Important management points and further investigations

Immediate management

Fluid resuscitation, including consideration of a urinary catheter, and a nasogastric tube are required ('drip and suck').

You should promptly involve your senior to discuss further management and imaging, which to some extent will depend on the cause and severity of the obstruction.

If there is evidence of perforation, you should involve your senior urgently as an operation will usually need to be performed.

Further management considerations

Seeking the cause is important as it will determine further management. In adhesional obstruction a trial of conservative management is usually indicated.

Further imaging

CT is more sensitive than plain films [1] and may demonstrate the cause.

Reference

[1] Nicolaou S, Kai B, Ho S, Su J, Ahamed K. Imaging of acute small bowel obstruction. Am J Roentgenol 2005;185:1036–44.

31 Gallstone ileus

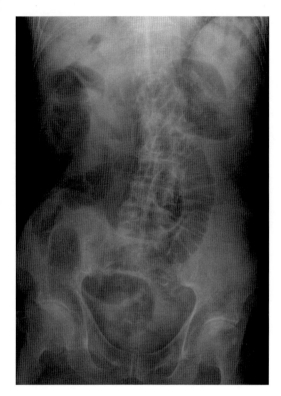

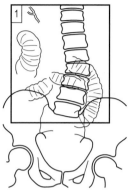

Fig. 31.1A This patient has gallstone ileus. This is a rare cause of small bowel obstruction but should always be sought on plain films as this is how the diagnosis is made.

Background

In gallstone ileus, the gallbladder adheres to the small bowel and a fistula forms between its lumen and the small bowel lumen. Stones from the gallbladder pass into the small bowel where they become impacted at the terminal ileum.

Clinical features

Clinical features are those of small bowel obstruction.

Radiological features

Remember that gallstones are only radio-opaque in 10% of cases but do look for them in the region of the terminal ileum. Not seeing a gallstone in the bowel does not exclude this diagnosis.

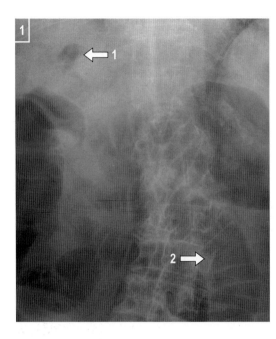

Fig. 31.1B Pneumobilia should be seen – look for air outlining the branching biliary tree (arrow 1). This air enters the biliary system from the duodenum (the biliary system normally contains no air). Air in the biliary tree occupies a central location within the liver and may resemble the trunk and central branches of a tree – this distinguishes it from portal venous gas where the gaseous lucencies are seen within the periphery of the liver and are generally finer in nature.

In gallstone ileus, pneumobilia will coexist with small bowel obstruction (arrow 2) (see Chapter 30).

Remember there are other causes of pneumobilia such as recent ERCP, and infection.

Important management points and further investigations

Immediate management

Immediate management is the same as for patients with small bowel obstruction. Operative management is required in these patients so involve your senior early.

This can be a difficult diagnosis to make – involve the radiologist, as they will also be performing the CT scan if it is required.

Further imaging

CT is the definitive modality. The stones will be more easily seen in the terminal ileum.

32 Large bowel obstruction

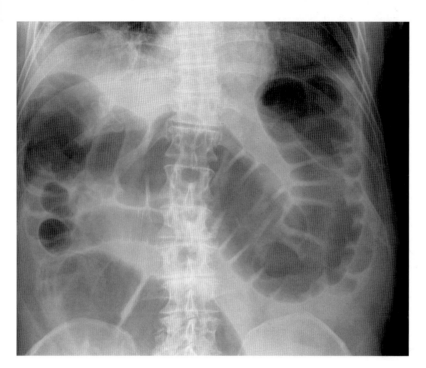

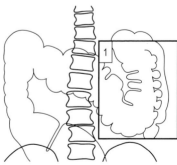

Fig. 32.1A This patient has large bowel obstruction, with dilated colon all the way to the mid descending colon. Note the incidental gallstones.

Background

Please read the section on small bowel obstruction as many of the points also apply here (Chapter 30).

Plain films are first line for diagnosis of large bowel obstruction although more complex investigations may be necessary to determine its cause.

Again, obstruction may be mechanical or functional. The commonest causes of mechanical obstruction are malignancy and diverticular disease. Volvulus is a less common, special form of obstruction which is discussed separately (Chapters 33 and 34). Pseudo-obstruction can affect the colon as well as small bowel and no plain film feature will differentiate the two conditions.

As in small bowel obstruction, look for evidence of perforation and remember to request an erect CXR.

Clinical features

Symptoms

Symptoms include colicky low abdominal pain, vomiting, absolute constipation and abdominal distension. Acute onset suggests a volvulus.

There may be symptoms preceding the obstruction that suggest an underlying tumour – weight loss, haematochezia, etc.

Signs

- Distended tympanic abdomen. Look for an abdominal mass.
- Peritonism may suggest perforation, which may complicate obstruction.

Differential diagnosis

- Small bowel obstruction – a radiological and clinical differential.
- Caecal volvulus and sigmoid volvulus have distinctive appearances on plain films.
- Inflammatory bowel disease with toxic megacolon (see Chapter 35).

A note on constipation

Constipation is a clinical diagnosis and is diagnosed by the finding of hard stool in the rectum on digital rectal examination. Constipation is not an indication for abdominal radiography.

Faecal loading is sometimes seen on abdominal films (see Fig. 32.2).

Radiological features

Tips for diagnosis of small bowel obstruction all apply here too, and the sequence of events is the same, although large bowel secretes less fluid than small bowel, so fluid-filled large bowel is a less common occurrence.

The key to diagnosis is to be familiar with anatomy. The position of much of the colon is fixed as much of the colon is retroperitoneal and thus fixed (ascending, descending and rectum).

The colon follows the periphery of the film, as opposed to small bowel which is central, and the transverse and sigmoid colon are the only parts which vary in position.

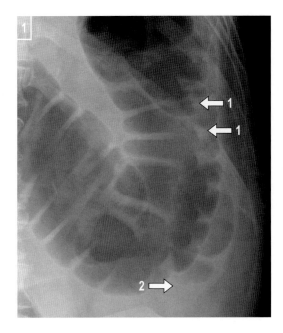

Fig. 32.1B The ability to differentiate between dilated small and large bowel is again important for interpretation. The large bowel in this radiograph is peripherally placed, as one would expect anatomically, and is dilated (>6 cm is considered obstructed).

The colonic haustrae do not traverse the entire diameter of the colon (arrows 1).

An abrupt change in colonic calibre may indicate the site of obstruction. This patient had a descending colonic carcinoma at endoscopy (arrow 2).

Always look at the diameter of the caecum as this is usually the point of rupture (>10 cm is worrying).

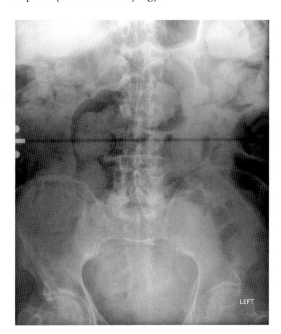

Fig. 32.2 Faecal loading. This is an appearance commonly seen on plain films. The stool in the colon appears mottled.

Important management points and further investigations

Immediate management

Fluid resuscitation, analgesia and a nasogastric tube are immediate considerations. Involve your senior in further management.

Further imaging

Differentiating between true mechanical large bowel obstruction caused by a tumour and pseudo-obstruction is very important as the former is usually treated operatively and the latter conservatively.

Once large bowel obstruction is diagnosed, the radiologist can perform either a diagnostic water-soluble contrast enema examination or a CT scan to determine the cause of the obstruction and help plan further management. The patient needs to be fairly mobile for the former procedure so a CT scan may be preferred in an immobile patient.

33 | Sigmoid volvulus

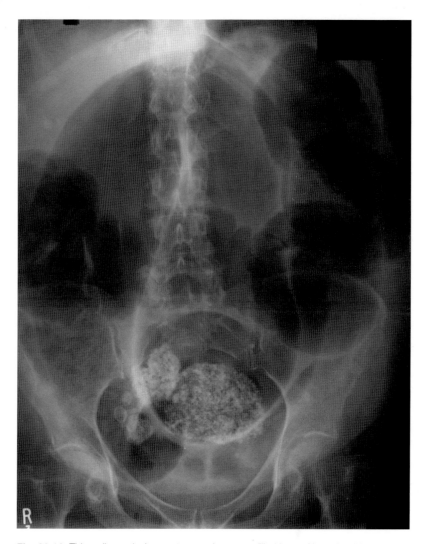

Fig. 33.1A This radiograph demonstrates a large gas-filled loop of bowel, arising from the left iliac fossa and pointing to the liver. It has a central sulcus giving it a coffee bean appearance. This is a sigmoid volvulus. The calcified densities in the pelvis are due to fibroids.

Background

This is a cause of large bowel obstruction, which results from the twisting of a long, redundant loop of sigmoid colon on its mesentery, causing proximal obstruction. It has a quite distinctive appearance on the plain radiograph, which is essential in the diagnostic pathway.

Patients with a long redundant sigmoid colon are at risk. These groups include elderly psychiatric patients and patients with chronic constipation who have been on long-term laxatives.

It is the commonest type of volvulus.

Clinical features

These can be rather non-specific but the condition can also present with acute large bowel obstruction – abdominal pain and a tympanic distended abdomen.

If not treated, it may lead to perforation and peritonitis.

Differential diagnosis

- Caecal volvulus can appear very similar (see Chapter 34).
- Sigmoid volvulus can also be confused with other causes of large bowel obstruction.

Radiological features

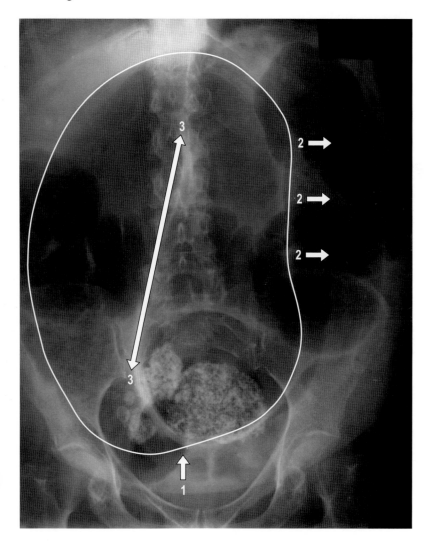

Fig. 33.1B Radiological features of sigmoid volvulus are as follows:
Gross distension of a gas-filled viscus in the central abdomen (outlined). A 'central sulcus' which gives the loop the appearance of a coffee bean (arrow 3). There is a sharp cut-off at the level of the pelvis (arrow 1). Because the twist is a loop of sigmoid colon, there is dilatation of the bowel immediately proximal to it: the descending colon (arrow 2). This is an important distinguishing feature from caecal volvulus where the small bowel is dilated. The loop points toward the liver.

Perform an erect CXR to rule out a perforation (see Chapter 27). Look for signs of perforation on an AXR also (see Chapter 45).

Important management points and further investigations

Immediate management

The radiographic appearances may be classic but a definitive test may need to be performed for confirmation.

Remember to resuscitate your patient with fluids/oxygen/nasogastric tube, etc.

Treatment is initially with a flatus tube. This may not work and in chronic cases, or in the presence of perforation, sigmoid resection may need to be considered.

Involve a general surgical team early.

Further imaging

Water-soluble contrast enema or contrast-enhanced CT may demonstrate the twist, and a 'bird beak' narrowing of the bowel at the level of the obstruction.

The duty radiologist may also help you with interpretation of the plain film.

34 Caecal volvulus

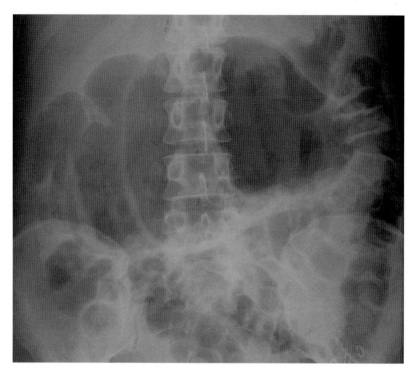

Fig. 34.1 This patient has a gas-filled caecum pointing towards the left upper quadrant of the abdomen. This is a caecal volvulus. (With thanks to Dr Maruti Kumaran for kindly providing this image.)

Background

Caecal volvulus is a rare but important condition, as it carries a high mortality rate.

It is caused by twisting of the caecum, which is often abnormally mobile in these patients, on its mesentery. The ascending colon is normally fixed and retroperitoneal. This leads to a closed loop obstruction, and rapid vascular compromise with resulting ischaemia and infarction.

Management is surgical and should be as prompt as possible.

Clinical features

There is acute colicky abdominal pain, and signs and symptoms of intestinal obstruction.

Patients are often young.

Differential diagnosis
- Sigmoid volvulus (Chapter 33).
- Gastric outlet obstruction (Chapter 29).

Radiological features
Caecal volvulus can be confused with sigmoid volvulus.
The plain abdominal x-ray is key for diagnosis.

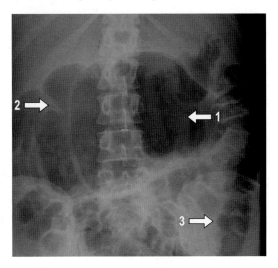

Fig. 34.2 This large gas-filled viscus (arrow 1) has the appearance of the caecum. It has haustrae that do not traverse the entire bowel (arrow 2). The obstructed caecum points towards the left upper quadrant (cf. sigmoid volvulus where the gas-filled sigmoid loop generally points toward the liver). Because of the twist occurring in the region of the caecum, dilated loops of small bowel are often seen and the distal colon is collapsed (arrow 3). Compare with sigmoid volvulus, where dilated colonic loops are seen (and the twist is in the distal sigmoid).

Very occasionally a dilated appendix may be seen arising from the caecum.

Important management points and further investigations
Immediate management
The patient may be very ill and should be made nil by mouth; an NG tube should be passed, and fluid resuscitation and analgesia administered.

This is a difficult diagnosis to make and plain film appearances are often not classic. Obtain your senior's help and that of a radiologist.

A prompt surgical opinion is advised.

Further imaging
CT may help to confirm the diagnosis.

35 Inflammatory bowel disease

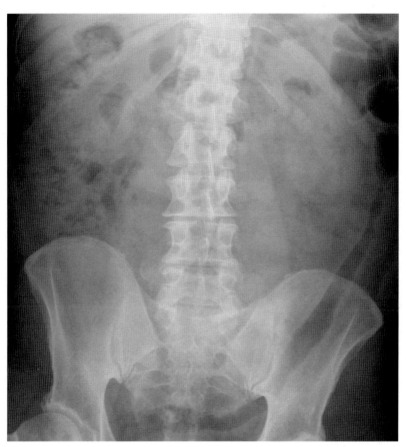

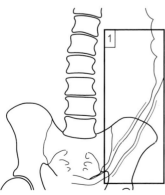

Fig. 35.1A This patient has thick-walled descending colon caused by active inflammatory bowel disease.

Background

Many conditions can cause the appearance of thick-walled bowel, with thumb printing.

The clinical presentation and patient demographics are important. This chapter aims to give an overview of all the conditions that produce this appearance on a plain film.

Inflammatory bowel disease refers to ulcerative colitis (UC) and Crohn's disease, which are of unknown aetiology. UC always affects the rectum and extends proximally, in a continuous manner. Crohn's disease can affect any part of the GI tract between mouth and anus with intervening normal segments, but terminal ileum is a common site.

Peak incidence for both conditions is in the second and third decades of life.

Toxic megacolon is a feared complication, which carries a high mortality rate. See below.

Clinical features

Symptoms

- Haematochezia
- Increased stool frequency, diarrhoea
- Abdominal pain
- Symptoms of extraintestinal manifestations (joint pains, iritis, rashes, perianal disease in Crohn's disease).

Signs

Signs include abdominal tenderness, pyrexia and tachycardia. The findings are non-specific.

These conditions can present to an on-call physician or surgeon as well as to A&E. The differentials can present on any ward – see below.

Differential diagnosis

Any of the following can cause the same appearances on plain radiographs. The clinical history is the key.

- Infective colitis (pseudomembranous colitis – *Clostridium difficile* infection in patients on broad-spectrum antibiotics. Patient will have an appropriate history and *Clostridium difficile* toxin will be present on the stool culture.)
- Ischaemic colitis – typically thick-walled bowel in the vascular 'watershed area' – splenic flexure.
- Typhlitis – in patients on chemotherapy; background history should make this clear.
- Lymphoma – causes thick-walled bowel; may not present acutely.

Radiological features

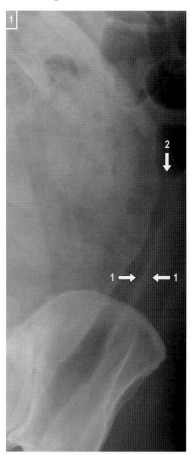

Fig. 35.1B The descending colon in this patient is thick walled due to mucosal oedema (arrows 1). Note the transition from thick-walled contracted bowel to normal calibre thin-walled bowel (arrow 2). There is loss of the normal haustral pattern in the diseased distal segment (lead pipe colon).

Thumb printing is a descriptive term to describe the appearance of thumb prints along the wall of the colon. It is actually due to thickened colonic haustrae. See Fig. 35.1C.

Look on the AXR for narrowed sacroiliac joints (often unilateral, or bilateral and asymmetric) as sacroiliitis is an extraintestinal manifestation of inflammatory bowel disease. They are normal in this patient.

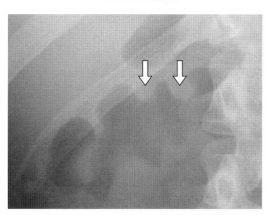

Fig. 35.1C This is a good example of thumb printing in a different patient (arrows).

Important management points and further investigations

Immediate management

Determine the cause (see above) – including taking a detailed history, sending stools for *Clostridium difficile* toxin and taking bloods.

Resuscitate the patient – fluid replacement is important. Consider antibiotics. Correct anaemia and electrolyte disturbance (hypokalaemia in diarrhoea).

Endoscopy is contraindicated in the acute setting because there is a high risk of perforation – a good reason for spotting the subtle abnormality on the plain film and thinking of the diagnosis.

Plain AXR may demonstrate thick-walled bowel and/or toxic megacolon. Serial AXRs are often performed to rule out developing toxic megacolon or to monitor its progress. Consider an erect CXR to rule out perforation (see Chapter 27).

This is not necessarily a diagnosis to rush your senior out of bed for but it is making the diagnosis that is the challenge, given that the clinical presentation can be non-specific. Toxic megacolon, however, is an emergency.

Further management considerations

Plain films are not particularly sensitive and consideration should be given to further imaging if the diagnosis is suspected.

Endoscopy and biopsy is necessary to make a firm diagnosis but this should be performed when the patient has recovered from their acute episode.

Once the diagnosis is confirmed medical therapy can be commenced.

Further imaging

- Consider serial films.
- CT can be helpful for diagnosis of complications.
- Small bowel contrast study or MR enteroclysis for Crohn's disease. Ultrasound can also be helpful.

Toxic megacolon

Toxic megacolon is a medical emergency. If this appearance is seen on an AXR senior input is required urgently.

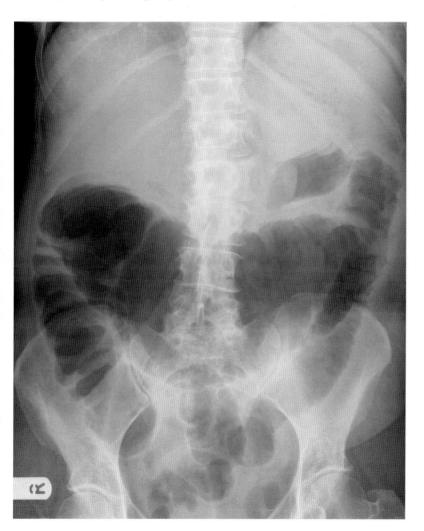

Fig. 35.2 This patient has a toxic megacolon. The whole colon is dilated. Over 6 cm is considered abnormal. Plain films are best for diagnosis. If it does not resolve in 24–48 hours, colectomy should be considered.

Note the thick-walled descending colon and thumb printing.

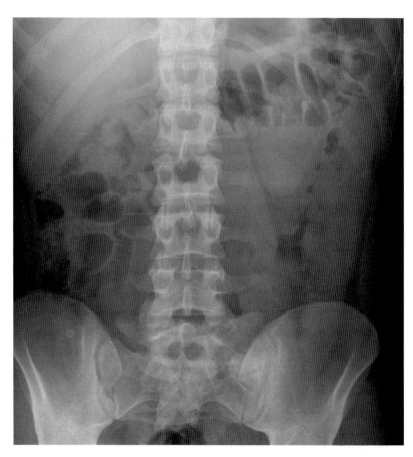

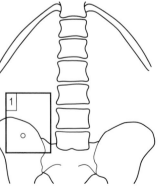

Fig. 36.1A This patient has a calcified density projected over the right ilium. This is an appendicolith in appendicitis.

Background

Appendicitis is one of the commonest surgical emergencies and can be a difficult diagnosis to make, as it can present in a variety of ways in a wide range of ages.

No single clinical finding, simple blood test or imaging modality can be used to reliably make the diagnosis, although US and CT are the best modalities where complex imaging is used. The AXR is not routinely indicated if appendicitis is suspected but it is useful to be aware of the AXR features if they are present in the patient who has undergone AXR for abdominal pain.

Clinical features

Appendicitis can present in several ways, classically with colicky central abdominal pain which migrates to the right iliac fossa and becomes worse on movement. Anorexia, fever and dysuria can be useful additional symptoms to elicit.

Signs include tenderness and rebound in the right iliac fossa (RIF), pain in the RIF on pressing the LIF (Rovsing sign), and tenderness on rectal examination (in a pelvic appendix).

Differential diagnosis

This is wide, particularly in young females, and includes:
- mesenteric adenitis and Meckel's diverticulum in children
- ovarian pathology, pelvic inflammatory disease and ectopic pregnancy in young females
- other conditions such as Crohn's disease, renal colic, urinary tract infection.

Radiological features

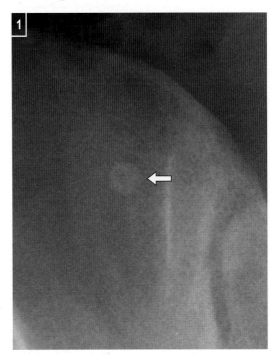

Fig. 36.1B The AXR is not sensitive or specific for appendicitis and should not be performed if the diagnosis is suspected. However, the finding of a calcified appendicolith in the RIF (arrow) is a relatively specific sign and should lead you to consider this diagnosis if you have not already done so. This is a relatively uncommon finding, seen in approximately 10% of patients with appendicitis.

Appendicitis is a relatively rare cause of small bowel obstruction, which may also be seen on the AXR; if the patient develops an appendix mass this may be seen in the RIF to be effacing bowel loops.

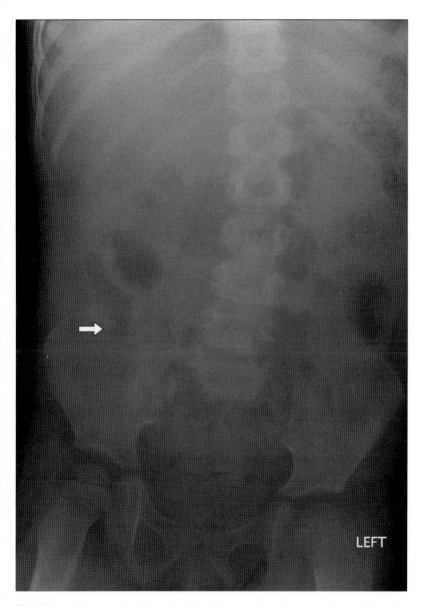

Fig. 36.2 This is appendicitis in a child, with the appendicolith once again seen (arrow).

Important management points and further investigations

Immediate management

Immediate surgical exploration is seldom indicated and observation may aid diagnosis. Keep the patient nil by mouth if this diagnosis is suspected and obtain a senior review.

Bloods including an FBC (for white cell count) and CRP may be helpful. Perform a pregnancy test in females of childbearing age.

Dip the urine for infection and blood.

Further imaging

This is not routinely indicated if the diagnosis is apparent clinically.

Compression ultrasound has high sensitivity and specificity, with an overall accuracy of about 85% in children. A normal ultrasound does not necessarily exclude appendicitis, but is almost always performed to exclude other causes of pain before performing an operation, particularly in young women, in whom there is a considerable differential diagnosis.

CT is also sensitive and specific but not routinely indicated.

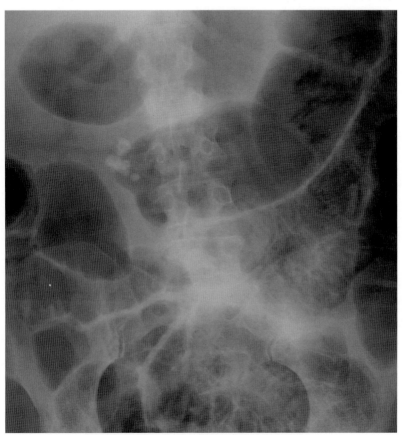

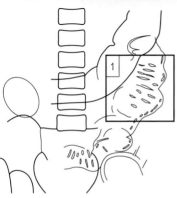

Fig. 37.1A This patient has extensive air in the bowel wall in the left lower quadrant of the abdomen which is in keeping with pneumatosis intestinalis. The patient had extensive bowel infarction.

Background

Pneumatosis intestinalis refers to air in the bowel wall, caused by ischaemia. Its presence implies impending perforation and it is an emergency. It often occurs in the setting of longstanding intestinal obstruction (see Chapter 30 & 32).

Consider this possibility in any very unwell, obstructed surgical patient. Such patients require a prompt operation. This condition carries a very high mortality rate.

Differential diagnosis

This condition should not be confused with pneumatosis coli, a benign condition caused by gas-filled vesicles in the colonic wall (see Fig. 37.2).

Radiological features

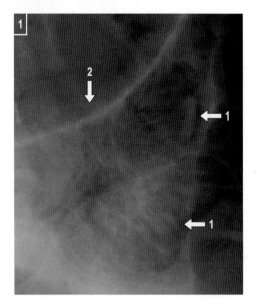

Fig. 37.1B There is air within the bowel wall giving the appearance surrounding the bowel wall seen on this radiograph (arrows 1).

This is due to ischaemic necrosis of the bowel wall and implies impending perforation. This appearance is not seen that often on a plain film but when seen it is an emergency.

In this case, the air in the bowel wall has assumed a linear configuration and involves small bowel loops and the caecum. This patient had experienced an embolism to the superior mesenteric artery following cardiac surgery with mitral valve replacement complicated by atrial fibrillation.

Compare with the normal colonic loop above (arrow 2).

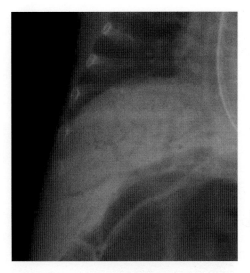

Fig. 37.1C Look carefully for air in branching portal vein radicles around the periphery of the liver which can also occur in mesenteric ischaemia (not present in this case). Portal vein gas is associated with a very poor prognosis in adults.

The image demonstrates the appearance of portal vein gas in a child.

Urgent CT can be performed if there is any doubt.

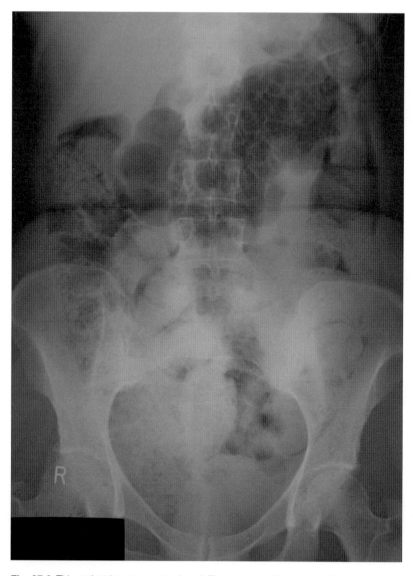

Fig. 37.2 This patient has pneumatosis coli. There are gas-filled cysts in the left upper quadrant. This is a benign condition. It does not follow the bowel wall. This condition is associated with COPD.

Important management points and further investigations

Immediate management

If you see this appearance, get your senior to promptly review the films and patient. You may need to consider a prompt operation so keep the patient nil by mouth and resuscitate.

Review old x-rays as worsening obstruction on these might make you more sure of the diagnosis.

Further imaging

This diagnosis is easier to make on a CT scan. However, detecting this abnormality on a plain film will help expedite urgent CT and optimal patient management.

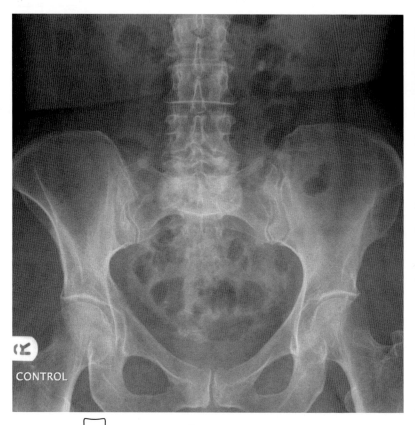

CONTROL

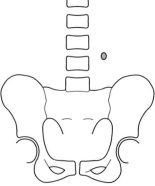

Fig. 38.1 This radiograph demonstrates an opacity to the left of the L3/4 disc space which represents a stone.

Background

Ninety per cent of urinary tract calculi are radio-opaque on a plain radiograph. There are several strategies for imaging suspected urinary tract calculi, which are described below.

Renal colic is a very common presentation to the on-call doctor. Infection proximal to obstruction is an emergency. Remember also that abdominal aortic aneurysms can present similarly.

Clinical features

Symptoms

There is acute loin pain, radiating to the groin. The onset of pain is usually sudden. Nausea and vomiting may also be a feature. The pain is visceral, so the patient is restless, and it is often the worst pain the patient has experienced.

Patients may have a prior history of urinary calculi.

It is important to ascertain whether the patient has signs and symptoms of infection such as pyrexia/rigors (as an obstructed infected kidney is an emergency) and whether they have a single kidney. Obstruction by a stone threatening the integrity of a single kidney is also an emergency which should be addressed immediately.

The patient may have frank or microscopic haematuria.

Signs

Loin tenderness is generally not a feature and suggests pyelonephritis.

Differential diagnosis

This is very wide and includes many causes of abdominal pain:
- pyelonephritis – usually insidious in onset; the patient is febrile, has loin tenderness on examination, and has leucocytes/nitrites/blood in urine
- appendicitis
- diverticulitis
- abdominal aortic aneurysm (Chapter 42) – ruptured or unruptured.

Radiological features

There are three methods for imaging suspected urinary tract calculi: plain radiographs, IVUs and unenhanced CT.

Plain radiographs

The traditional first line was to obtain a plain radiograph, centred on the urinary tract – a 'KUB' film (kidneys, ureters, bladder).

It is still useful to be able to assess such a film for ureteric calculi, as you may also detect a ureteric calculus in a patient presenting on the surgical 'take' with abdominal pain. But this is now not the first-line investigation if stones are suspected.

A knowledge of the course of the ureter is important for proper assessment of a plain film of the abdomen (see Chapter 28).

Any calcific density along the course of the ureter should be considered as a potential ureteric stone.

Phleboliths – small calcifications in the pelvic small vessels – can be confused with stones but they are generally completely round, and have lucent centres.

The intravenous urogram

Intravenous urograms (IVUs) have been superseded by CT in most centres, but in some hospitals they are still the first line for diagnosis of ureteric calculi. This is generally the only indication for an out-of-hours IVU.

Intravenous contrast is injected into the patient (see the section on CT and contrast risks, p. 9). This is concentrated by the kidneys and excreted into the pelvicalyceal (PC) systems and ureters after about 5 minutes. It shows up white on a plain radiograph. IVUs involve taking serial films after injection of contrast. A limited on-call series might be as follows:

- A control film is taken to look for calcifications. Subsequent films are compared to this.
- A film performed at 10–15 minutes will capture the contrast in the PC systems and ureters. If it looks as though excretion is delayed on one side, further films can be taken until the level of obstruction is established. This can be a lengthy process in high-grade obstruction and may take several hours.
- One way of deciding when to take delayed films is to take the first at 30 minutes then double the interval each time until the study is complete.
- A post-micturition film is taken which may confirm obstruction.

You are looking for evidence of a calculus on the control film. Most calculi cause a degree of obstruction, which is demonstrated by delayed excretion of contrast on the side of the obstruction and dilatation of the PC system and ureter on that side. Contrast is often held up on the side of the obstruction.

Figs 38.2–38.4 show an example.

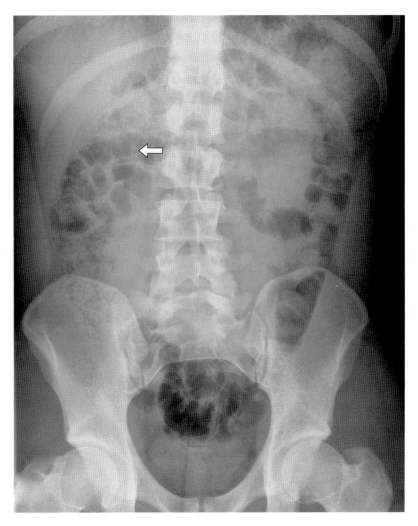

Fig. 38.2 This control film in a patient with a suspected right renal stone shows an opacity (arrow) suspicious for a stone. It is difficult to be certain because of overlying bowel.

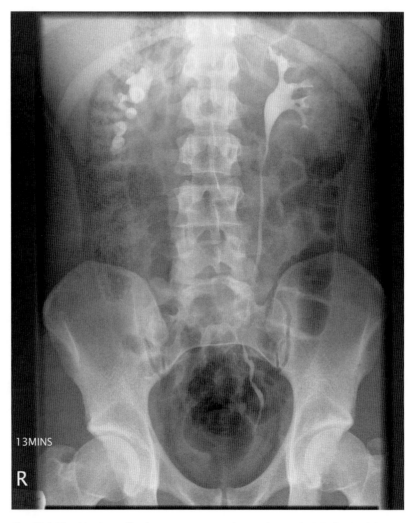

Fig. 38.3 The 13-minute film demonstrates normal excretion on the left. On the right the PC system is dilated. Contrast has not yet reached the opacity so a delayed film is performed.

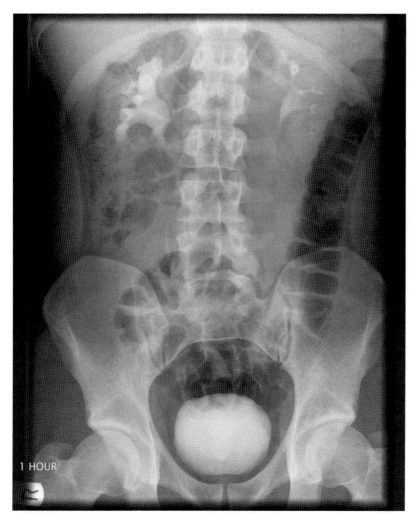

Fig. 38.4 The one-hour delayed film now shows contrast up to the point of the opacity. The IVU has demonstrated obstruction caused by a proximal calculus at the right pelviureteric junction (PUJ). Calculi are commonly seen at the PUJ or the vesicoureteric junction (VUJ) at the point where the ureter enters the bladder.

Imaging with CT

Unenhanced CT (sometimes known as a CTKUB, CT kidneys, ureters, bladder) is now the gold standard in most hospitals. It is more sensitive than IVU and does not usually require the use of intravenous contrast. It can also diagnose alternative causes of pain.

Important management points and further investigations

Immediate management

- Analgesia, particularly with non steroidal anti-inflammatory agents. Remember that these are nephrotoxic, so check the U+E beforehand.
- Refer to urology once the diagnosis has been confirmed.
- If the patient has an obstructed infected kidney, urgent nephrostomy may need to be considered and this should be decided by a urologist in consultation with an interventional radiologist.
- If the patient has a single obstructed kidney, this may also be an indication for an emergency nephrostomy.

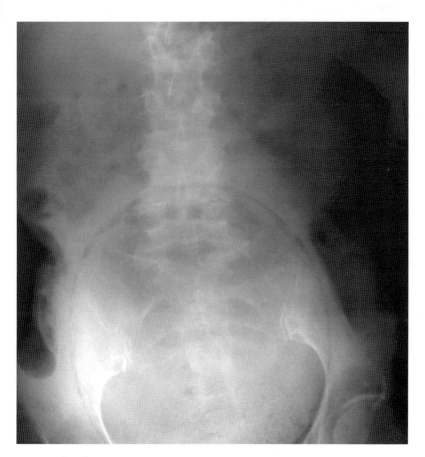

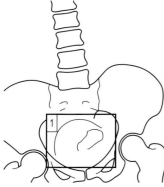

Fig. 39.1A This radiograph demonstrates air in the bladder wall. These appearances are consistent with emphysematous cystitis. (With acknowledgement to Dr Gill Markham for providing this radiograph.)

Background

This condition has the same aetiology as emphysematous pyelonephritis (Chapter 40). It is commoner in patients with diabetes and is caused by gas-forming organisms. It has a high untreated mortality rate, and the plain film may be the only available clue to this diagnosis.

Clinical features

Symptoms

- Symptoms of urinary sepsis – dysuria, frequency, etc.
- The patient may have diabetes.

Signs

There may be signs of infection (fever, tachycardia, hypotension).

Differential diagnosis

Lower or upper urinary tract infection.

Radiological features

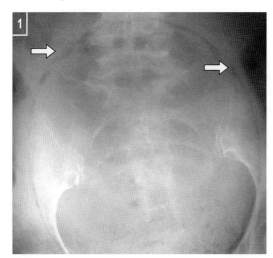

Fig. 39.1B These patients have air in the bladder wall. The pathological process is similar to patients with emphysematous pyelonephritis. The air is caused by gas-forming organisms.

The diagnosis is based upon the anatomical location of the air – which corresponds to the bladder wall (arrows).

Important management points and further investigations

Immediate management

- Patients should be commenced on appropriate antibiotic therapy. Liaise with the microbiology department for advice on appropriate antimicrobial selection.
- Fluid resuscitation may be necessary; these patients are usually unwell.
- A urology opinion may be helpful.

Further imaging

If the diagnosis is unclear, a non-contrast CT scan of the bladder will help to localize the air.

40 Emphysematous pyelonephritis

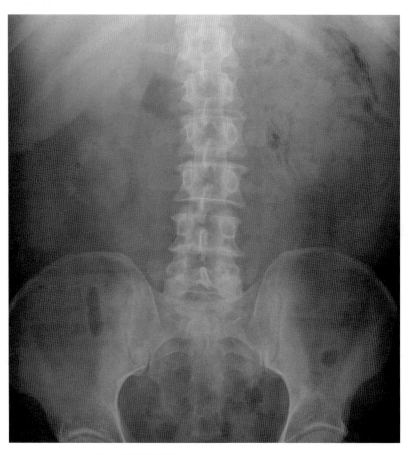

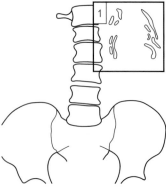

Fig. 40.1A This patient has abnormal air in the region of the left kidney. These are the appearances of emphysematous pyelonephritis.

Background

This is a rare but life-threatening condition, with a reported mortality of about 40% [1]. If you recognize the radiological features promptly and start the right treatment you could save a life.

The condition is caused by gas-forming organisms that give rise to an upper urinary tract infection. It is commoner in people with diabetes and can be associated with renal calculi.

It can coexist with emphysematous cystitis (see Chapter 39).

Clinical features

Symptoms

- Symptoms of pyelonephritis (fever, abdominal pain, nausea and vomiting)
- Patients may present with acute renal failure.

Signs

- Pyrexia
- Loin tenderness.

Differential diagnosis

Clinical features are not specific. This is a radiological diagnosis.

Radiological features

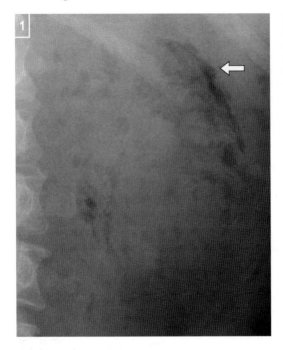

Fig. 40.1B This patient has abnormal gas shadows surrounding the left renal outline (arrow). These are caused by gas-forming organisms in the left kidney.

Important management points and further investigations

Immediate management

- Resuscitation measures and intravenous antibiotics should be administered promptly. Remember to check renal function/FBC as thrombocytopenia and renal impairment are associated with a poor outcome.
- Perform blood cultures.
- Urgent urology opinion is advised.
- Nephrectomy may need to be considered.

Further imaging

CT is the gold standard and may help to demonstrate stones.

References

[1] Wan YL, Lo SK, Bullard MJ, Chang PL, Lee TY. Predictors of outcome in emphysematous pyelonephritis. J Urol 1998;159(2):369–73.

41 Chronic pancreatitis

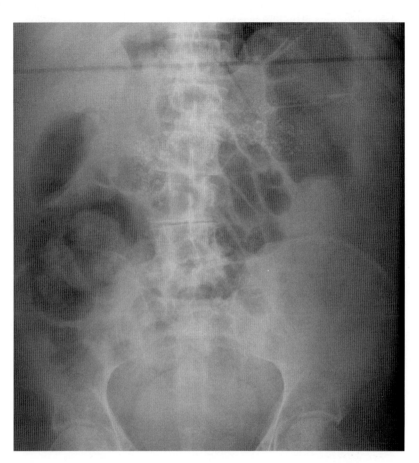

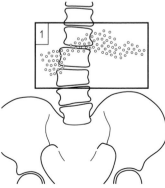

Fig. 41.1A There are punctate calcifications throughout the pancreas, due to chronic pancreatitis.

Background

Chronic pancreatitis is not an emergency per se, but the finding of pancreatic calcifications on a plain film may help you make this diagnosis in a patient presenting with severe abdominal pain.

It is most commonly caused by alcohol, although gallstones are amongst the several other causes of this condition. It results in an atrophic gland with calcifications. Diagnosis is often delayed so suspecting it clinically and spotting it on the radiographs may make a difference to management of your patient. Approximately 4% of these patients go on to develop pancreatic cancer after 20 years.

Clinical features

Symptoms

There is severe recurrent abdominal pain, vomiting, diarrhoea and weight loss.

Signs

These are non-specific.

Differential diagnosis

- Any cause of an acute abdomen, in particular acute pancreatitis.
- Acute pancreatitis can present on a background of chronic pancreatitis.

Radiological features

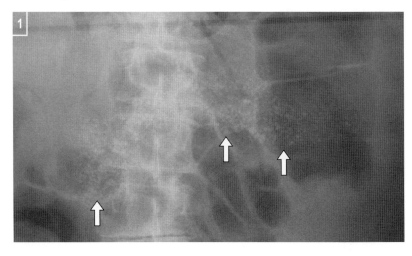

Fig. 41.1B Punctate calcification in the pancreas is seen in approximately 30% of cases but is quite specific if seen (arrows).

Awareness of the anatomy of the pancreas is key for diagnosis. The pancreas is comma-shaped and located at the level of the L1–L2 disc space.

Important management points and further investigations
Immediate management
Pain relief will be required. This is not normally a life-threatening condition.

Further imaging
CT may confirm pancreatic atrophy and demonstrates calcifications well.
ERCP/MRCP may demonstrate beading of the pancreatic duct but they do not show calcifications.

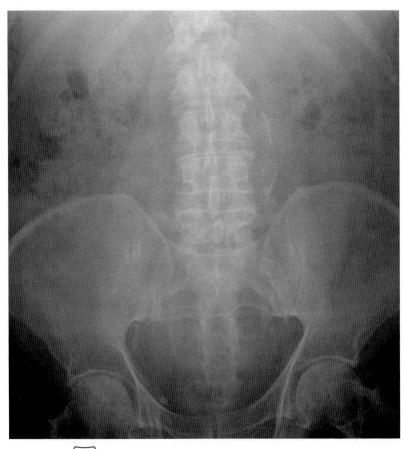

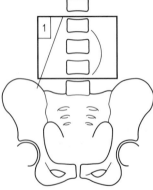

Fig. 42.1A This radiograph demonstrates a calcified abdominal aortic aneurysm (AAA). The psoas shadow is lost on the left, suggesting a rupture.

Background

AAA is a common cause of death in elderly patients, with men being affected more than women. The overall mortality is about 50% in ruptured aneurysm and many die before reaching hospital.

The best predictor of rupture is maximum aneurysm diameter: as this increases, the risk of rupture increases. Aneurysms above 5 cm in diameter have a high risk of rupture – those measuring 5–6 cm have a 3–15% annual risk, whereas those over 8 cm have a 30–50% risk. Always look at previous imaging if available when this diagnosis is suspected or made.

Plain radiography is NOT the first investigation to request if this diagnosis is suspected, as it is not very sensitive or specific for the presence of an AAA. However, many patients presenting with abdominal pain have an AXR performed as part of their investigative work-up. When interpreting any plain AXR, the presence of a calcified AAA should always be checked for. If the features are present on the radiograph (often unexpectedly), immediate action is required.

Think of this diagnosis in every patient presenting with abdominal pain. It is a diagnosis not to be missed, and the presenting features (see below) are rather non-specific. You may save a patient's life.

Clinical features

Symptoms

Unruptured

- Can be asymptomatic (up to 75%)
- Back pain.

Ruptured

- Severe, sudden-onset abdominal and back pain
- Syncope
- Vomiting; haematemesis if complicated by aortoenteric fistula.

Signs

There is an expansile mass in the abdomen, which will be tender if the aneurysm has ruptured. Hypotension is also a sign of rupture.

Patients may have concomitant atherosclerotic disease (ischaemic heart disease, renal disease, hypertension, cerebrovascular disease, limb ischaemia).

The patient may present to the general/vascular surgeon on call, A&E, or the medical team.

Differential diagnosis

The presenting symptoms of a symptomatic aneurysm, ruptured or unruptured, are non-specific. Therefore the list of differential diagnoses is wide. Renal colic and acute back problems are acute presentations that are also non-specific and may cause particular confusion.

Radiological features

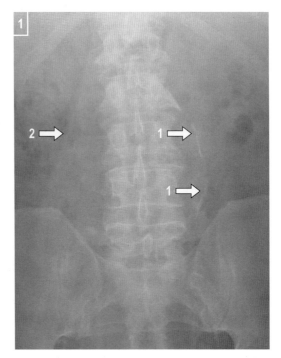

Fig. 42.1B The convex outline of a calcified AAA can be seen in the midline in about 75% of cases (arrows 1). Sometimes the aneurysm is non-calcified and a very subtle convex outline should be sought.

The psoas outline should be sought (see p. 146). This is lost if there is retroperitoneal pathology. When an aneurysm ruptures, blood pools adjacent to the psoas muscle in the retroperitoneum. Blood is the same radiographic density as muscle, so the psoas outline is obliterated (silhouette sign, p. 4–5). Here the left psoas shadow is lost suggesting a ruptured aneurysm, whereas the right psoas shadow can be more clearly seen (arrow 2). It should be remembered that loss of the psoas outline can be a normal finding, especially on the right. This sign is therefore non-specific. It is important to correlate radiological findings with clinical presentation and indices.

Important management points and further investigations

Immediate management

If an aneurysm is seen on the plain AXR, establish if it is ruptured (see signs and symptoms above) whilst stabilizing the patient. You should **involve your senior early** in the management of these patients.

  If the aneurysm is thought to be clinically ruptured, involve the vascular surgeon.

Remember ABC in the management of an acutely unstable patient:
- Airway should be secured.
- Breathing – oxygen and saturation monitoring.
- Circulation – Two large-bore intravenous cannulae should be inserted and bloods taken including FBC, U+E, clotting screen, amylase and cross-match (inform the blood bank as O negative may be required before type-specific blood is available). The white cell count may be raised in ruptured aneurysm.

A urinary catheter should also be placed and analgesia administered.

Inform ITU/anaesthetics as a bed may need to be arranged if operative management is required.

See further imaging below.

Further management considerations

If the AAA is unruptured, the patient should be followed up by the vascular team, usually in the outpatient setting.

Further imaging

To reiterate, an AXR is NOT part of the work-up for a patient with a suspected AAA. However, you may detect an AAA on an AXR performed for other reasons, which will prompt the management steps outlined above.

If the patient is stable, CT with intravenous contrast may be helpful. This will help to establish the correct diagnosis (presence of aneurysm versus other pathology, and presence of rupture). CT will also help to determine if the patient is suitable for an endovascular repair (EVAR).

The unstable patient may need to be transferred immediately to theatre. Portable ultrasound can be helpful to determine the presence or absence of an aneurysm while resuscitation takes place although this should not delay definitive management. Ultrasound is not sensitive for diagnosis of rupture.

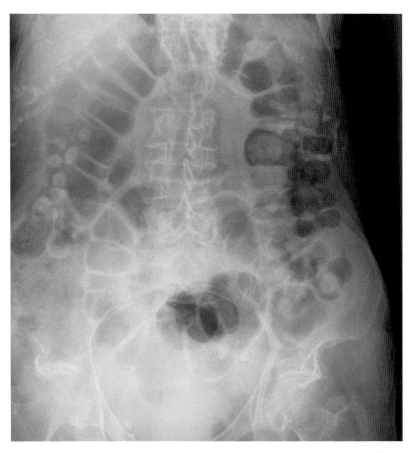

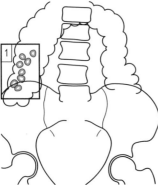

Figure 43.1A This patient has gallstones in the right upper quadrant. Note the faecal loading in the colon.

Background

Gallstones are sometimes seen incidentally on plain films. Plain films are not requested specifically to look for gallstones as they are only radio-opaque in 10% of patients – ultrasound is the first line if they are suspected. But gallstones may be seen if a plain film is included in the work-up of a patient with abdominal pain, and they may be the cause of the patient's presentation.

Biliary colic, cholecystitis, gallstone ileus and acute pancreatitis are all acute presentations that may be associated with gallstones.

Radiological features

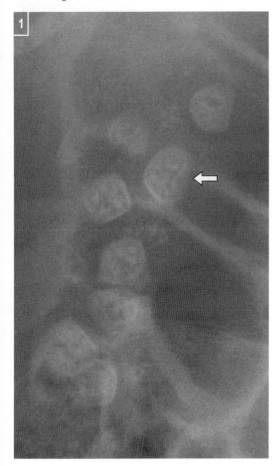

Fig. 43.1B Ten per cent of gallstones are radio-opaque (arrow).

Think of the diagnosis if you see calcifications in the right upper quadrant. Remember that renal stones can also be seen in the same region but will always be projected over the right kidney (see Chapter 38).

Gallstones may be lamellated or multifaceted as in this case. They are also generally larger than renal stones.

Important management points and further investigations

Immediate management

Consider whether the stones are causing the patient's presentation. Administer analgesia. Perform blood tests including liver function tests and amylase to rule out pancreatitis.

Further management considerations

A surgical review may be helpful.

Further imaging

An ultrasound may be helpful for confirmation and to examine the biliary tree.

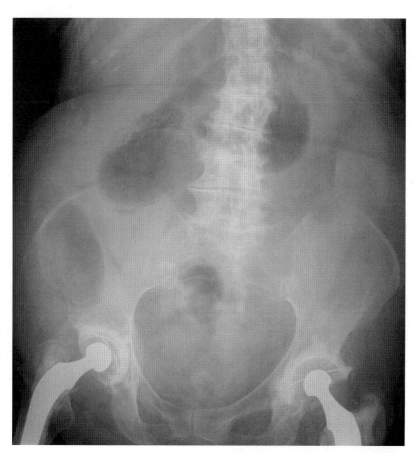

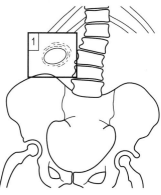

Fig. 44.1A This patient has a dilated viscus with surrounding punctate air in its wall. The CT scan confirmed emphysematous cholecystitis. Note the hip replacements and severe degenerative changes in the spine. (With thanks to Dr J.C. Jobling for kindly providing the radiograph.)

Background

This refers to infection of the gallbladder with gas-forming organisms. It is a rare condition but carries a high mortality, in the region of 20%. It is commoner in elderly males and tends to be associated with diabetes.

The gallbladder can perforate as a complication.

Clinical features

Symptoms and signs are similar to those of acute cholecystitis, with right upper quadrant pain and tenderness which may be accompanied by fever and tachycardia.

Gallbladder perforation may lead to peritonitis.

Radiological features

The plain film is not the gold standard for diagnosis but the classic findings on the plain radiograph should prompt urgent action.

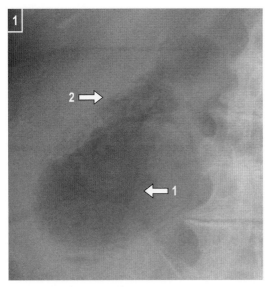

Fig. 44.1B This rounded viscus is a rather low-lying gallbladder (arrow 1). The finding of punctate air bubbles in the wall of any viscus should prompt alarm (see Chapters 37, 39, 40) and the gallbladder is no exception. Here, punctate air bubbles are seen surrounding the gallbladder wall – the hallmark of emphysematous cholecystitis (arrow 2). Do not confuse this appearance with faeces or air in the colon (Chapters 32 and 37).

Important management points and further investigations

Immediate management

Emphysematous cholecystitis is an emergency. Discuss with your senior and a general surgeon if it is suspected.

Prompt antibiotic treatment should be instigated but this does not constitute definitive treatment. These patients generally require either radiological drainage or surgery. For this reason keep the patient nil by mouth. Intravenous access and fluid resuscitation are important.

Further imaging

CT is the gold standard to confirm the diagnosis and to diagnose perforation if present.

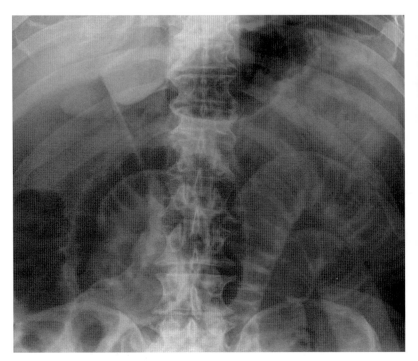

Fig. 45.1A Large pneumoperitoneum.

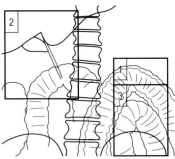

Background

Please see Chapter 27 for an account of perforation on an erect CXR.

The diagnosis of pneumoperitoneum is more difficult to make on an AXR than a CXR. However, if it is suspected, both an erect CXR and supine AXR should be performed as an erect CXR is only 80% sensitive for perforation and an AXR may provide further information. AXR is, however, only about 50% sensitive for perforation.

The AXR may also reveal the cause of the perforation, for example obstruction.

Clinical features

Please see Chapter 27.

Radiological features

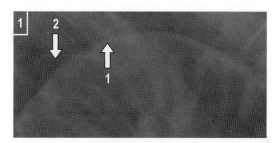

Fig. 45.1B *Rigler's sign:* On a normal AXR, all air is contained within the bowel lumen. Thus it only outlines the **luminal surface** of the bowel (arrow 1), The luminal surface of the bowel can be seen because of the difference in density between air and bowel wall (see Introductory section, p. 3).

When a viscus perforates, there is air within the peritoneal cavity which can now outline the **outside** of the bowel wall (arrow 2). This is known as Rigler's sign, where both sides of the bowel wall are seen.

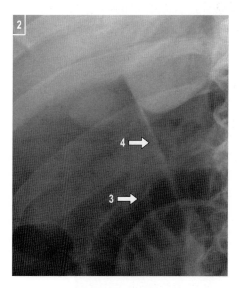

Fig. 45.1C Arrow 3 shows bowel **without** Rigler's sign for comparison in which only the luminal surface is outlined by air.

Silverman's sign: The falciform ligament is not usually seen on a normal AXR as it is of soft tissue density. In patients with pneumoperitoneum, air can collect on both sides of it, outlining it and it is seen as a diagonal line in its expected anatomical position (arrow 4).

211

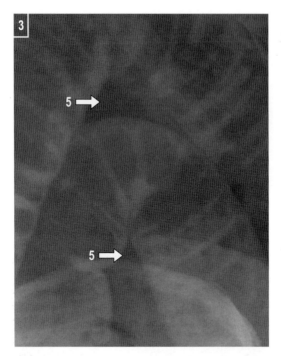

Fig. 45.1D *Lucent liver sign:* The liver is normally of soft tissue density. Air can collect anteriorly over the liver in pneumoperitoneum giving it a darker hue.

Triangles of air: These are abnormal. There are no normal triangular structures in the abdomen in which air can collect. Kinked loops of bowel provide triangular spaces in which air can collect. Suspect perforation when triangles are seen (arrows 5).

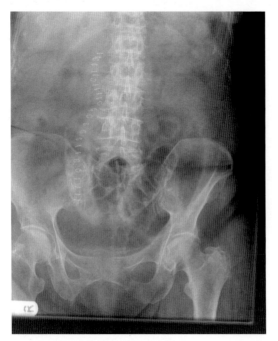

Fig. 45.2 Football sign: usually seen in babies, a very large perforation can collect anteriorly on an AXR (the patient is supine), producing a large, round gas shadow. Rigler's sign is also present in this case.

Important management points

See Chapter 27.

This can be a difficult diagnosis to make. Involve your senior and/or radiologist early. The stakes are high – you must get it right as a patient with a pneumoperitoneum will usually require a laparotomy.

Further imaging

A left lateral decubitus film, taken with the patient lying on their left side, will allow air to accumulate superiorly in the right flank, aiding diagnosis. This can be used in patients who are too unwell to sit upright for an erect radiograph, or in babies who cannot sit upright (Fig. 45.3). The left lateral position is chosen to avoid diagnostic confusion when interpreting the film. If the film was taken with the patient on their right side then the left lung base (which is lower than the right) may obscure free air or air in the gastric fundus may mimic it (see p. 138).

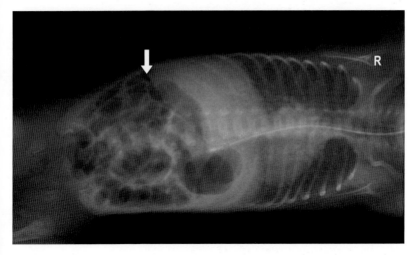

Fig. 45.3 A lateral decubitus film in a baby. Air has collected around the liver (arrow), confirming a perforated viscus. (This is a rather subtle example).

Further imaging with CT can be considered in equivocal cases as CT is highly sensitive, and considered the gold standard for confirming perforation, although it will not necessarily identify the cause.

Further reading

Earls JP, Dachman AH, Colon E, Garrett M, Molloy M. Prevalence and duration of postoperative pneumoperitoneum: sensitiviy of CT versus left lateral decubitus radiography. Am J Roentgenol 1993;161:781–5.

Levine MS, Scheiner JD, Rubesin SE, Laufer I, Herlinger H. Diagnosis of pneumoperitoneum on supine abdominal radiographs. Am J Roentgenol 1991;156:731–5.

Bone x-rays

Fractures

Other

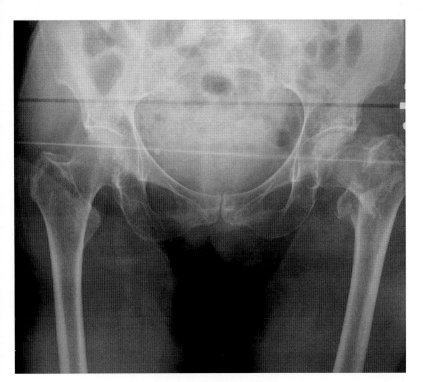

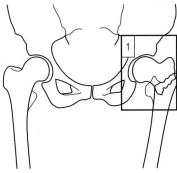

Fig. 46.1A There is a sclerotic line traversing the left hip, which represents an intertrochanteric fracture.

Background

This is an important fracture in the ward scenario, often suffered by osteoporotic patients who fall out of bed, and prompt diagnosis is essential. It may also be encountered by on-call junior doctors who may be asked to review the patient following a fall. They may be unfamiliar with how to investigate and refer such a patient. This chapter is intended to help the junior doctor make this diagnosis and to make an appropriate referral.

Patients presenting with hip fractures may also present to A&E or orthopaedics.

Fractures are usually radiolucent (dark on the radiograph) lines traversing bone. Also look for a breach of the cortex, and discontinuity of linear bone trabeculae. If a fracture is impacted look for a sclerotic (white on the radiograph) line traversing the bone – this does not intuitively look like a fracture but in the correct clinical setting should be correctly interpreted as such.

Always get two views if you can (in this case an AP pelvis and lateral hip). A fracture may be completely invisible on one view and obvious on the other.

Clinical features

The patient has hip pain following a fall, and the leg on the side of the fracture is shortened and externally rotated. A patient with a femoral fracture is unlikely to be weight-bearing, although some patients can walk (albeit painfully) on an impacted femoral neck fracture.

Radiological features

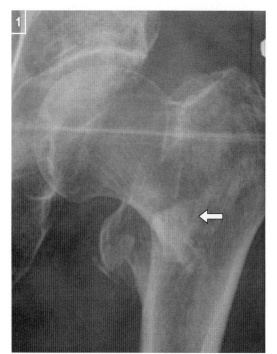

Fig. 46.1B This is an example of the impacted type of fracture. The fracture line is sclerotic in this case, because of overlapping bone fragments (arrow).

Also look for pelvic fractures, particularly of the pubic rami, as these can present very similarly to a femoral neck fracture.

Remember to request and look at a lateral film. If the fracture is obviously seen on the AP, though, and the patient cannot raise their leg for the lateral there is no need to insist that one is taken.

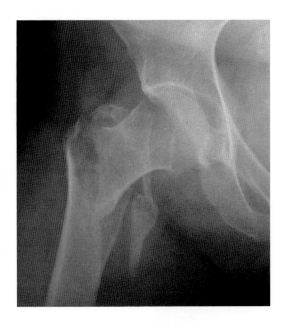

Fig. 46.2 This radiograph of a different patient demonstrates a lucent line traversing the intertrochanteric region. This is the commoner appearance of a hip fracture.

Important management points and further investigations

Immediate management

Remember simple measures such as analgesia.

If you are confident of the diagnosis clinically, remember that the patient is likely to undergo prompt fixation so consider performing a CXR if the patient has respiratory or cardiac disease as part of the anaesthetic work-up.

And if the fracture is confirmed, referral to orthopaedics, nil by mouth, group and save/clotting/FBC, etc. will be needed.

The site of the fracture determines the type of operation. The hip capsule provides the blood supply to the femoral head so a very proximal fracture of the neck requires a hemiarthroplasty. Fractures more distally (intertrochanteric and subtrochanteric) are generally fixed with screws.

Further imaging

A hip fracture may be present but may be completely invisible on a plain film. Interval radiographs, or MRI may be necessary to make the diagnosis. Ask a radiologist if you are unsure.

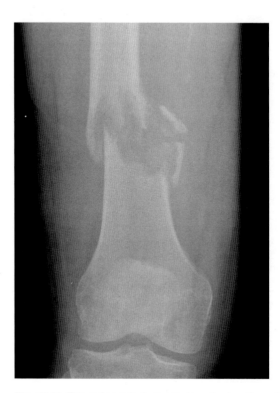
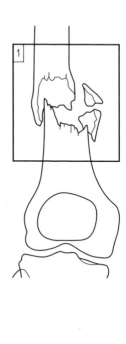

Fig. 47.1A This radiograph demonstrates a fracture through an aggressive lesion in the distal femoral diaphysis. This is a pathological fracture through a lytic metastasis.

Background

Please read the sections on benign versus aggressive lesions (Chapter 49) and bone metastases (Chapter 53).

This is a scenario that often causes confusion, hence its inclusion in this book.

A pathological fracture occurs in a bone that is weakened by a pathological process. This is usually a tumour, which may be a primary or secondary, but can also be infection. The process need not necessarily be a malignant or aggressive one – benign lytic lesions of bone can also fracture.

This condition might be expected to present to an orthopaedic or A&E doctor but many of the processes that weaken bone can occur on a medical ward too.

Also be aware that preventative measures can be taken to prevent fractures of bones with lytic metastases – consider an orthopaedic opinion before the bone breaks, particularly if it is a weight-bearing one.

Clinical features

Signs and symptoms are those of a fracture but the amount of trauma will be less than that normally expected to fracture a bone.

Differential diagnosis

A non-pathological fracture.

Radiological features

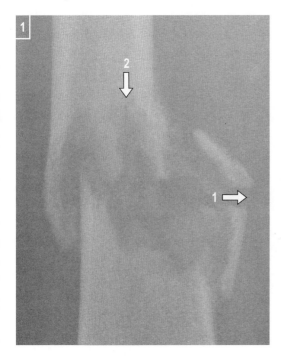

Fig. 47.1B There is a lytic lesion in the bone which has fractured (arrow 1). See the wide zone of transition (arrow 2) and compare with aggressive bone lesions (Chapter 49).

This is clearly not a simple fracture. However, comminution in simple fractures can cause confusion.

Important management points and further investigations

Immediate management

Refer to an orthopaedic surgeon. Management of these cases is complex but should include immobilization and analgesia to reduce pain. Diagnosis may require biopsy. A sample can be taken during fixation.

Further imaging

Review the CXR if done to see if there is a tumour. If the primary tumour is not known, discuss further imaging with a radiologist.

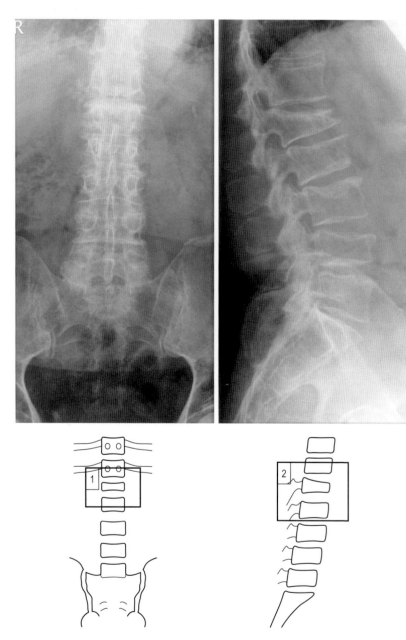

Fig. 48.1A Lateral (left) and anteroposterior (right) views of the lumbar spine demonstrating loss of anterior height of the L1 vertebra in keeping with a wedge compression fracture.

Background

Wedge compression fractures have a range of aetiologies. The commonest presentation to the on-call ward doctor is the osteoporotic wedge compression fracture. This chapter will help you to diagnose this condition.

Fractures secondary to trauma can also have this appearance – these patients usually present to the emergency department. Lumbar spine trauma is not covered in detail here.

The other causes of wedge compression fractures are myeloma and metastatic disease to the vertebra. These are pathological fractures (see Chapter 47). They can be difficult to distinguish from osteoporotic fractures but the clinical presentation may be a clue – known malignancy or symptoms of such, and multiple compression fractures in abnormal looking bones, in an unusual non-weight-bearing distribution.

MRI is sometimes needed to distinguish between the two.

Clinical features

There is usually localized back pain. Examine carefully for neurology – this mandates an MRI. Some wedge compression fractures may be asymptomatic.

Radiological features

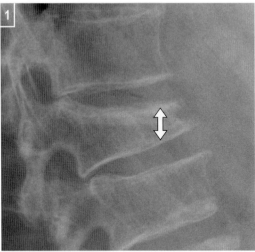

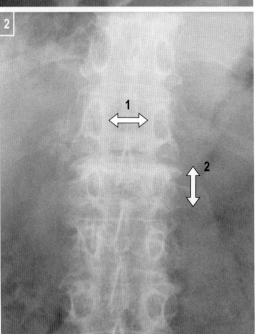

Fig. 48.1B On the lateral film (top image), a wedge compression fracture will demonstrate loss of anterior height (arrow). The anterior part of the vertebral body should be the same height as the posterior part. Look at the background density of the bones. If all are osteopenic, as here, the aetiology of the fracture may be osteoporosis. Also look at the density of the vertebra in question and whether any of it has been destroyed to suggest a malignant aetiology.

The pedicles on an AP film (lower image) may be important in distinguishing malignant from benign collapse: the pedicles appear round, at the lateral aspects of each vertebral body (arrow). If a pedicle is lost, this is suggestive of a malignant aetiology involving the posterior elements of the vertebra. Osteoporotic collapse generally involves the vertebral body and not the pedicles.

Fig. 48.1B caption continued

On the AP film, the vertebral body may demonstrate loss of overall height (arrow 2). This is not demonstrated in Fig. 48.1B (lower image) because the height of the posterior aspect of the vertebral body is preserved. It is generally seen in advanced cases in which there is global loss of height of the vertebra.

An end-stage collapsed vertebra is linear and flat – sometimes called a 'vertebra plana'. Wedge compression fractures are often multiple – consider imaging the whole spine.

Important management points and further investigations

Immediate management

Osteoporotic collapses are rarely associated with neurological symptoms and signs, and can generally be managed conservatively, with analgesia and measures to increase bone density in the longer term. However, it is sometimes difficult to be confident that a collapsed vertebra is definitely due to osteoporosis, even in the absence of such signs and symptoms and MRI may need to be considered in these patients.

A malignant collapse is more frequently associated with neurological signs and symptoms which may be rapidly progressive. There may be clues such as weight loss, a known diagnosis of cancer as well as clues on the film as described above.

If there are neurological symptoms and signs, an urgent spinal or orthopaedic opinion is advised with a view to MRI imaging. Spinal cord compression is an emergency which mandates prompt operative management or radiotherapy to prevent permanent deficit.

Further imaging

MRI as detailed above may be helpful, to diagnose the cause of neurology or to establish if the collapses are malignant.

If malignancy is suspected, a CXR may diagnose a lung primary, and staging CT may be required.

The following table of x-rays summarizes features of benign and aggressive lytic (destructive) processes in bone. These are areas of increased lucency in bone. Remember that aggressive processes include infection as well as tumour (see Chapters 50 and 53).

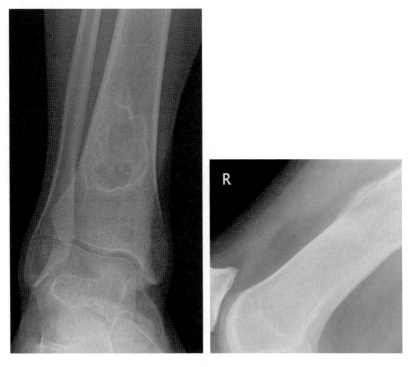

Fig. 49.1 Examples of benign (left) and malignant/aggressive (right) processes in bone.

	Benign	**Aggressive**
	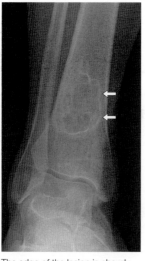	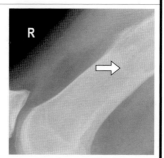 The edge of the lesion in an aggressive lesion is poorly defined (arrow). It almost blends into the surrounding bone. This is referred to as a wide zone of transition. Sometimes the abnormality is multifocal or permeative and the bone appears moth eaten. This is also an aggressive pattern.
Edge/ zone of transition	The edge of the lesion is sharply defined and may be sclerotic – of higher density – as in this case (arrows). The edge of the lesion can be referred to as the zone of transition.	
	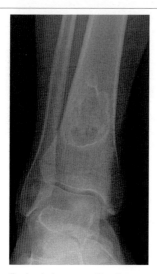	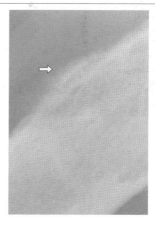 Aggressive lesions may have periosteal reaction with a less organized appearance and this may have the appearance of sunburst (spiculated) or lamellar (layered) reaction (arrow). This is an acute periosteal reaction which has not had a chance to organize itself.
Periosteal reaction	Benign lesions may either have no periosteal reaction, or smooth periosteal reaction, such as in a healing fracture.	

	Benign	Aggressive
Cortical destruction	Benign lesions do not usually destroy the cortex, but may be expansile and cause thinning or scalloping of cortex (particularly on the endosteal aspect of the cortex).	Malignant lesions may destroy the cortex, as seen at the superior aspect of this lesion, where the femoral cortex is lost.

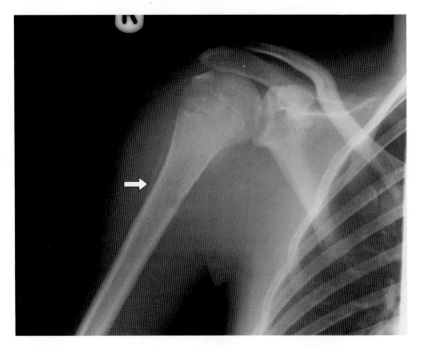

Fig. 49.2 This is an osteosarcoma in a teenager – another example of an aggressive process. It has a permeative appearance which is ill-defined in the proximal humerus with marked periosteal reaction on both sides of the proximal humerus (arrow).

Further reading

Helms CA. Fundamentals of skeletal radiology. 3rd ed. Edinburgh: Elsevier; 2004.

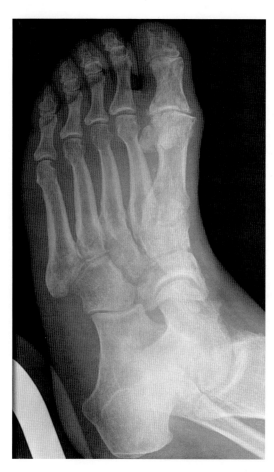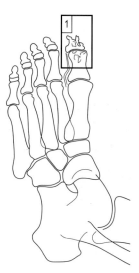

Fig. 50.1A This patient has osteomyelitis of the left great toe, particularly affecting the distal phalanx.

Background

The main routes of bone infection (osteomyelitis) are either haematogenous or direct. Haematogenous osteomyelitis is commonest in children. Situations in which direct routes may occur include infected ulcers in diabetic patients, and post-surgery (especially with metalwork) and as a sequela of an open fracture.

Clinical features

Symptoms

- Fever and local pain
- The foot is a common site when there is a direct route of infection such as an ulcer in a person with diabetes.

Signs

- Tenderness and pyrexia
- An overlying non-healing ulcer or sinus in a diabetic patient
- Local erythema and restricted movement.

It is important to be aware of this condition as it may present to several different groups of junior doctors. It may present to orthopaedics, particularly in patients at risk such as those who are post-surgical or who have suffered an open fracture.

These patients may also present to a general medical team (particularly diabetes and endocrinology) or vascular team.

Differential diagnosis

Septic arthritis if near a joint.

Radiological features

Osteomyelitis is an example of an aggressive bone lesion (see Chapter 49).

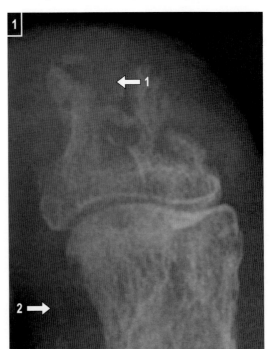

Fig. 50.1B Osteomyelitic bone has the appearance of a lucent lesion or several lucent lesions in the bone (arrow 1). It can affect any part of the bone. The bone in this example looks moth eaten. The edge of the lesion is ill defined – this is referred to as a wide zone of transition and is a feature of an aggressive bone lesion.

Also note the calcified digital artery in this diabetic patient (arrow 2) – a clue to diagnosis.

Look at the overlying soft tissue, as swelling may be the earliest sign (not present in Fig. 50.1B). There may also be periosteal reaction (also not present in Fig. 50.1B). See Chapter 49 for an example.

Remember that the radiographic changes may lag behind the clinical presentation.

Any aggressive process in bone can appear similar. The site is often a clue – metastases seldom occur in the very distal appendicular skeleton. And the clinical presentation should guide you. This patient had an ischaemic ulcer on their great toe – direct inoculation of infection.

In patients with prostheses and metalwork look for lucency near the metalwork to suggest infection.

Important management points and further investigations

Immediate management

Request bloods including inflammatory markers and a full blood count, and blood cultures.

Intravenous antibiotics (often a long course is required) and referral to an orthopaedic team for further management.

Further management considerations

Plain films are not particularly sensitive and consideration should be given to further imaging if the diagnosis is suspected.

Further imaging

A three-phase bone scan is the most sensitive modality. MRI is also very sensitive.

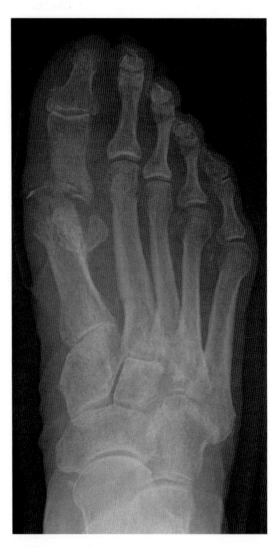
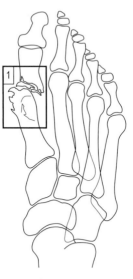

Fig. 51.1A This radiograph demonstrates a destructive erosive process involving the first metatarsophalangeal joint with associated subluxation of the joint. This patient has septic arthritis.

Background

Septic arthritis refers to infection of a joint. It can occur in several different patient groups: in adults post-joint replacement, post-traumatically or spontaneously, especially in diabetics. Another important patient group is the limping child with a septic hip (see discussion in Chapter 59, 'Perthes' disease').

It is important to make the diagnosis as early as possible. Patients may become very ill and delayed or missed diagnosis may lead to destruction of the joint, a particular issue in children.

Clinical features

The condition usually presents as a monoarthritis of sudden onset. It may be caused by septicaemia. Elicit a history of joint replacement or trauma. There may be signs and symptoms of infection – fever, unwellness, joint pain and effusion.

In children – septic arthritis, Perthes' disease, slipped upper femoral epiphysis (SUFE) and irritable hip need to be differentiated. Always think of infection, which can occur at any age. Irritable hip is a diagnosis of exclusion and other possible causes must be excluded before this diagnosis is made.

Age is the key discriminator. SUFE most commonly occurs in 10–16-year-olds (see Chapter 58) and Perthes' disease in children aged 5–12 (see Chapter 59). These patients are usually systemically well. Irritable hip occurs in children aged 3–10. There is usually a preceding or concomitant viral illness. Systemic pyrexia is unusual.

One study [1] demonstrated that paediatric patients who were non-weight-bearing, with erythrocyte sedimentation rate (ESR) > 40, white cell count $>12 \times 10^9/L$ and fever almost always had septic arthritis.

Differential diagnosis

- Any monoarthritis (e.g. gout)
- Osteomyelitis (Chapter 50).

Children:

- Perthes' disease
- Slipped upper femoral epiphysis
- Irritable hip.

Radiological features

Plain film radiology has a limited role as the changes occur late in the natural history of the disease. However, identification of key features is very important.

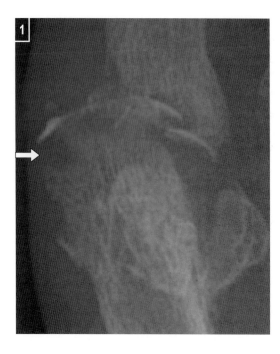

Fig. 51.1B Several large joint erosions are seen (arrow). These show aggressive features (Chapter 49). Look for lucency. There may be associated soft tissue swelling.

This patient's joint is also subluxed.

Do not rely on radiography. The diagnosis is generally made using other modalities.

Important management points and further investigations

Immediate management

This presentation is an emergency. A CRP/ESR/FBC should be performed (see above). Joint ultrasound can be considered to look for an effusion – aspiration of joint fluid with microscopy (to look for crystals – which are seen in gout/pseudogout, which are important differential diagnoses) and Gram staining/culture. MRI may also be helpful.

Consider antibiotic therapy, particularly if a joint aspiration is negative for crystals.

Prompt senior review and orthopaedic referral are required in these cases.

Further management considerations

Prosthetic joints are very difficult; the diagnosis is not easy to make and the stakes are high: antibiotic treatment is likely to be ineffective with the prosthesis in situ but revision is a major undertaking. Comparison with old films may help: look for radiolucency around the prosthetic components of the joint and/or subperiosteal new bone formation that are new findings.

Further imaging

* As above
* A three-phase bone scan can be helpful for diagnosis of prosthetic infection.

Reference

[1] Kocher MS, Mandiga R, Zurakowski D, et al. Validation of a clinical prediction rule for the differentiation between septic arthritis and transient synovitis of the hip in children. J Bone Joint Surg 2004;86-A(8):1629–35.

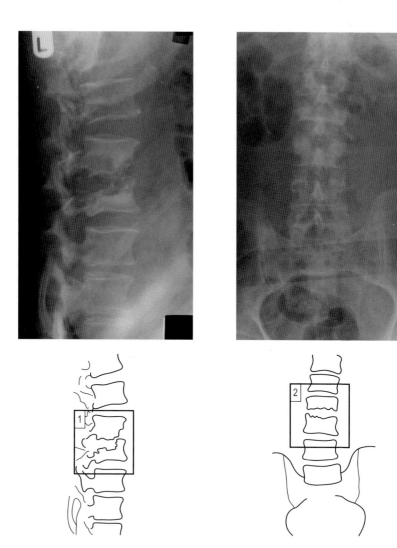

Fig. 52.1A These lateral and AP radiographs of the lumbar spine demonstrate destruction of the L2/L3 disc space caused by discitis.

Background

Discitis refers to infection of the intervertebral disc. It is an important condition with a relatively high mortality rate, in the region of 5%. It can affect children and adults, the peak age being 50.

Discitis can occur postoperatively or spread to the disc haematogenously. *Staphylococcus aureus* is a common pathogen. TB (tuberculous discitis) is another common cause, particularly in certain ethnic groups.

Clinical features

Onset may be insidious and clinical features non-specific, especially in tuberculous discitis.

Symptoms

Symptoms include localized back pain and fever.

Signs

There is localized tenderness. There may also be a neurological deficit.

Radiological features

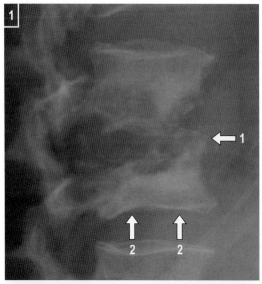

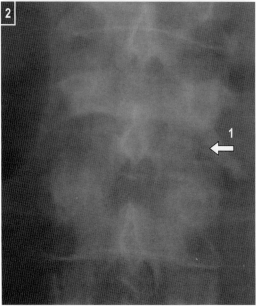

Fig. 52.1B Radiographic changes in discitis on a lumbar spine film occur relatively late and may not be evident for several weeks from the onset of disease. If there is a strong clinical suspicion, an MRI scan should be performed.

However, be vigilant for the signs on a plain film, as the radiographic signs may be present when the diagnosis was not considered clinically. The earliest sign is disc space narrowing.

This becomes associated with lucency of the adjacent endplates, caused by bone destruction and calcification of the disc.

In later discitis, as in this case, the endplates are destroyed (arrow 1). Compare the smooth edge of a normal vertebral body endplate (arrows 2).

Important management points and further investigations

Immediate management

This is a relative emergency. An early orthopaedic/spinal opinion is advised if this diagnosis is suspected, even if the plain film is normal.

Blood tests should be performed: high inflammatory markers raises suspicion.

Early antibiotic therapy should be considered.

Further imaging

MRI is the gold standard and can detect associated soft tissue complications such as abscesses. CT and bone scintigraphy can also help to make the diagnosis.

53 Bone metastases

Background

Bone metastases are aggressive lesions (see Chapter 49). It is important to detect them as their presence will have an impact on further management.

Always look at the bones, on any plain radiograph (this includes CXR, AXR etc.), for bone metastases.

Bone metastases may present with bone pain, or be asymptomatic. They may present as a pathological fracture (see Chapter 47).

Radiological features

Bone metastases may be lytic (lucent), sclerotic (increased density) or mixed (elements of lytic and sclerotic). These properties can be used to help determine the tumour of origin if this is not known:

- lytic metastases: causes include lung, breast, renal cell, thyroid and bowel cancer, melanoma, myeloma and lymphoma
- sclerotic metastases: causes include prostate cancer
- mixed metastases: causes include breast cancer.

Bone metastases can have a wide variety of appearances and this account is not exhaustive.

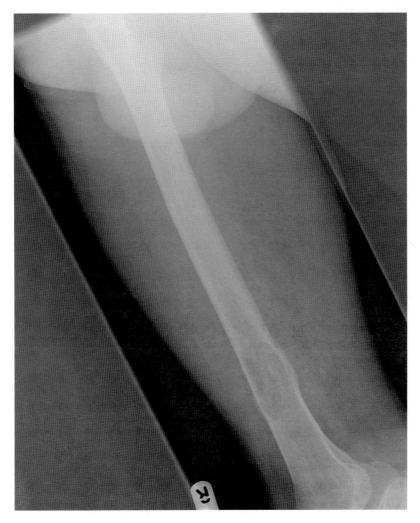

Fig. 53.1 Bone metastasis. This patient has a lytic metastasis in the distal femur. The primary tumour in this case was lung cancer. Note the aggressive features (see Chapter 49).

Remember that metastases weaken bone and that this patient is at risk of a pathological fracture. Refer to orthopaedics for prophylactic pinning before this happens.

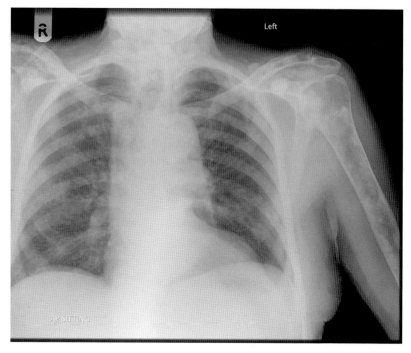

Fig. 53.2 Sclerotic bone metastases. This patient has several sclerotic metastases involving all of the visualized bones. The patient had prostate cancer (the breast shadow on the left is due to gynaecomastia).

Sclerotic metastases can be more difficult to distinguish from benign sclerotic lesions. The zone of transition is wide – this is an important feature.

Important management points and further investigations
Immediate management

This is not an emergency situation which requires immediate action but spotting this abnormality can alter a patient's management.

Remember that if a weight-bearing bone is affected all the way through the cortex, this is a fracture risk.

Further management considerations

- The primary tumour may be known, or hitherto undiagnosed.
- Clinical examination and a thorough history are required.
- Examine the breasts, prostate; perform a rectal examination.
- Look at the CXR if this has been done for a lung tumour or lung metastases.
- Remember myeloma – organize urine electrophoresis.
- An ultrasound or CT scan may be considered to diagnose the primary.
- A bone scan may determine the site of other metastases.

54 Gas gangrene

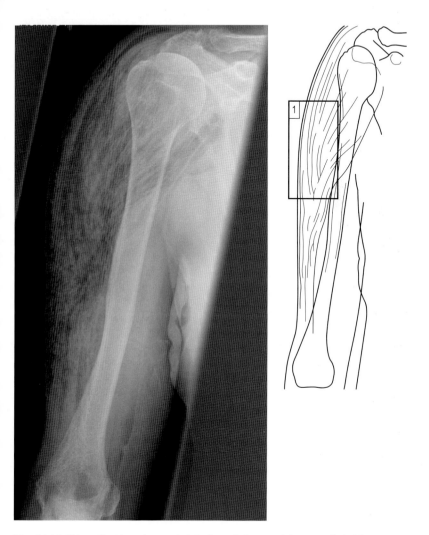

Fig. 54.1A This patient has abnormal air in the soft tissues of the upper limb. These appearances are due to gas gangrene.

Background

Gas gangrene is caused by gas-forming organisms (*Clostridium* species) infecting muscle and soft tissue; this often occurs by direct inoculation into the muscle but can also spread haematogenously. The condition is rapidly fatal and is often recognized too late for treatment, which involves surgical debridement.

It may present to physicians, surgeons, A&E doctors or orthopaedic surgeons. Those who are diabetic or immunocompromised are at risk. Mortality is in the 25–100% range.

Clinical features

Symptoms

- Severe pain out of proportion to the signs is suggestive of gas gangrene.
- Gas gangrene may progress rapidly over hours.

Signs

- Initially the skin may be yellow in colour, with local crepitus.
- Skin necrosis may be a feature.
- Signs of toxaemia may be present: fever, tachycardia and hypotension.

Differential diagnosis

Cellulitis – are the symptoms out of proportion to the signs? If so consider gas gangrene.

Radiological features

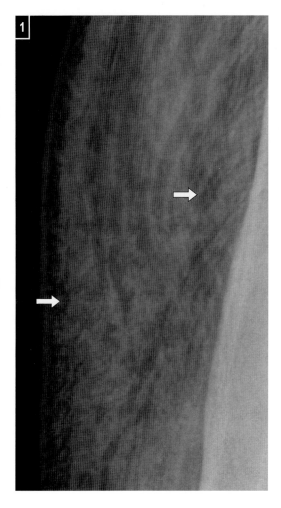

Fig. 54.1B The plain film findings are of air in the soft tissues in the area of interest. This is not a specific finding; it can accompany such conditions as fractures and pneumothorax.

In the correct clinical context this finding should be taken very seriously.

This patient has extensive air over the soft tissues of the upper limb (arrows). An amputation saved this patient's life.

Important management points and further investigations

Immediate management

If suspected call your senior immediately. This condition can kill within hours. An urgent surgical opinion is advised. Start intravenous fluids and make the patient nil by mouth to prepare for theatre. Don't forget analgesia.

Further management considerations

These patients require extensive debridement or amputation.

Further imaging

CT is particularly sensitive for subcutaneous air as well as giving information about the extent of involvement, but do not let it delay definitive management.

Paediatric x-rays

This section includes a range of conditions that may be encountered by the junior doctor working on-call in paediatrics, or in the emergency department in paediatrics. We have excluded neonatal conditions, which are normally not managed by the on-call junior doctor, and fractures.

Many paediatric conditions have already been described in the adult chapters, with examples and explanations of how they differ in children.

Please see the following chapters:

Chest

Abdomen

Bones

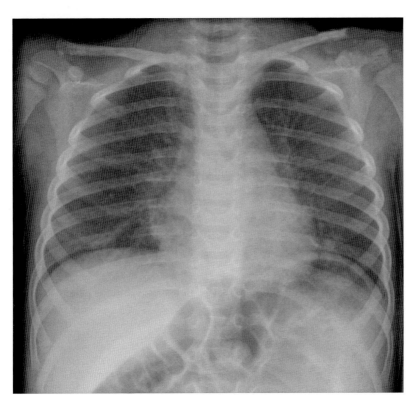

Fig. 55.1A This young child has increased peribronchial markings in both lungs, indicative of a viral pneumonia.

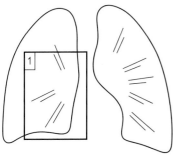

Background

A viral aetiology for pneumonia is particularly common in children although it can also occur in adults.

Viral pneumonia has a different pattern to bacterial pneumonia on a CXR. The CXR appearances of viral pneumonias are generally non-specific but certain appearances can suggest the diagnosis.

Children generally develop a mild self-limiting illness. Respiratory syncytial virus (RSV), adenovirus and influenza are common causes in children.

See also Chapter 8.

Clinical features

Symptoms

These include shortness of breath and upper respiratory tract symptoms – coryza, cough, sore throat.

Signs

Fever and wheeze are the main signs. There may also be a viral maculopapular rash.

Radiological features

CXR features of viral pneumonias may be non-specific but the pattern is different from bacterial pneumonia.

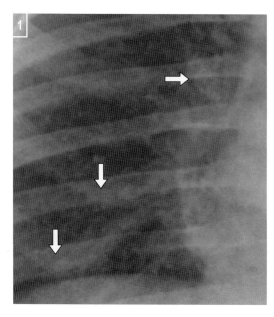

Fig. 55.1B The CXR demonstrates increased bronchovascular markings throughout the lungs (arrows), due to thickening of the bronchial walls.

Changes in viral pneumonias tend to be interstitial in pattern (lines) rather than alveolar (consolidation pattern).

In younger children with viral lower respiratory tract infection, mucus plugging of bronchi can cause segmental or lobar areas of collapse (see Chapter 17).

Important management points and further investigations

Immediate management

Management is usually supportive. Consider oxygen therapy and antipyretics, and observe closely. Monitor oxygen saturation with pulse oximetry.

Further imaging

This is not usually required.

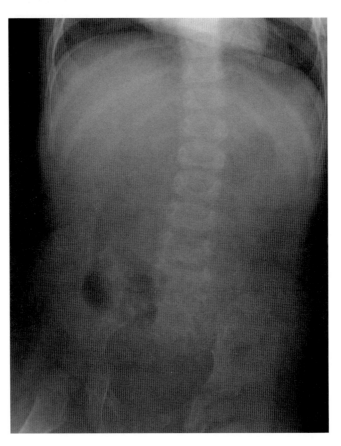

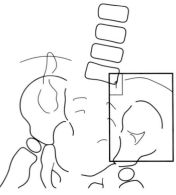

Fig. 56.1A This figure demonstrates a very subtle soft tissue mass protruding into the bowel lumen – this abnormality is projected over the left side of the pelvis. This proved to be an intussusception.

Background

This condition is caused by telescoping of one section of bowel (the intussus-ceptum) into an adjacent section (the intussuscipiens). This commonly occurs in the terminal ileum. There can be a pathological lead point (commoner in adults) or it can occur spontaneously (commoner in children, 90% of cases).

The condition usually occurs in infants aged 3–12 months although it can occur later than this and is commoner in boys.

Clinical features

Symptoms

- Abdominal pain. The pain may be intermittent and lead to the legs being drawn up.
- Redcurrant jelly stools may occur.
- Vomiting.

Signs

- Abdominal mass
- Fever.

Radiological features

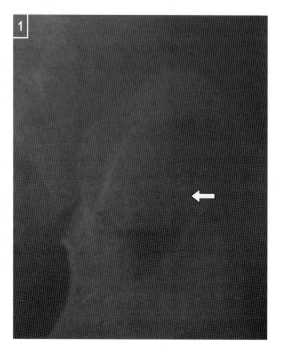

Fig. 56.1B This patient has a soft tissue mass protruding into the large bowel. It is subtle (arrow). There may be signs of obstruction proximal to the level of the intussusception. The mass may be evident as a lack of bowel loops in that area.

Sometimes air may be seen trapped alongside the bowel which has telescoped. Look also for signs of perforation, which is a rare complication.

Plain films are not the best modality for diagnosis but will often be the first one you see. Picking up the subtle signs may prompt you to request an ultrasound, which is more sensitive.

Important management points and further investigations
Immediate management

Management includes resuscitation with fluids, nil by mouth, analgesia and senior review. Blood tests should also be done. Faecal occult blood testing may help to confirm the presence of blood.

Consider arranging an ultrasound.

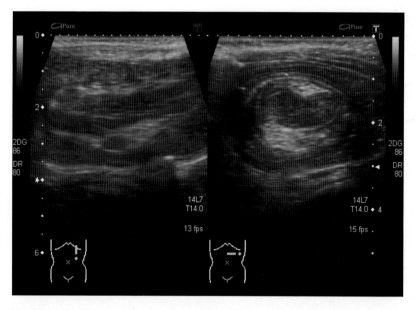

Fig. 56.2 Ultrasound from the same patient showing that there is an abnormality at the site arrowed in Fig. 56.1B. This shows telescoping in longitudinal section (left) and a target sign in transverse section (right).

Further imaging

Ultrasound may help confirm the diagnosis.

A therapeutic air or contrast reduction enema is the first-line treatment unless contraindicated (perforation). It can also be used for diagnosis. This requires discussion with both a specialist radiologist and paediatric surgeon (as perforation is a complication which requires surgical treatment). Air reduction is not appropriate if ultrasound demonstrates a pathological lead point for the intussusception (e.g. duplication cyst of the bowel) or is suggestive of bowel necrosis.

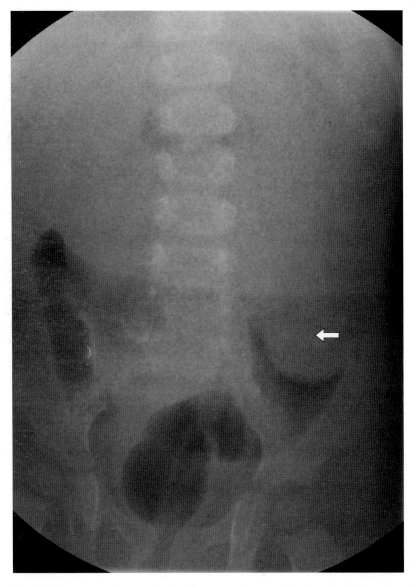

Fig. 56.3 An air reduction showing the intussusception more clearly on the left (arrow).

57 Retropharyngeal abscess

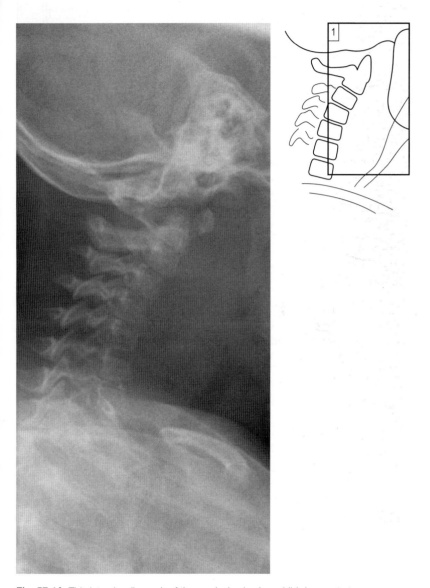

Fig. 57.1A This lateral radiograph of the cervical spine in a child demonstrates gross increase in the soft tissue in the retropharyngeal space, effacing and displacing the trachea anteriorly. The child had a retropharyngeal abscess.

Background

An abscess in the retropharyngeal space is associated with high morbidity and mortality in children, particularly if not detected early. It may complicate upper respiratory tract infection, or be a complication of local trauma, for example from ingested foreign bodies.

The most feared complication is loss of the airway, although there is significant associated morbidity from mediastinitis, vascular compromise and epidural abscesses.

Clinical features

Symptoms

The chief symptoms are sore throat, fever, difficulty and pain on swallowing, and neck stiffness.

A history of trauma to the area can be trivial and may be forgotten.

Signs

Drooling and/or stridor are worrying signs of potential airway compromise. Cervical lymphadenopathy is also commonly seen.

If epiglottitis is being considered, it can be potentially dangerous to examine the throat as this can compromise the airway.

Differential diagnosis

Acute epiglottitis is a similar emergency condition caused by bacterial infection and swelling of the epiglottis which can rapidly compromise the airway. The history is often shorter, and the child will often be drooling with dysphagia and respiratory distress. Epiglottitis can compromise the child's airway even more quickly than retropharyngeal abscess and in both conditions if there are signs of airway compromise this must be addressed before any consideration of imaging.

Radiological features

A lateral cervical spine radiograph, assuming the airway has been secured, may help make the diagnosis.

CT is more sensitive but carries a higher radiation dose.

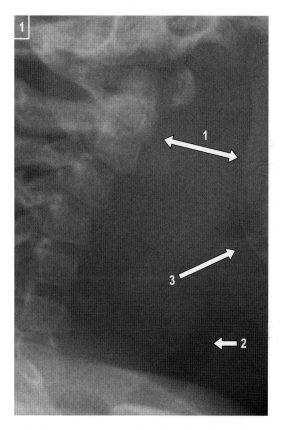

Fig 57.1B The retropharyngeal space on a lateral cervical spine radiograph is seen behind the air-filled trachea and pharynx. Increased prevertebral soft tissue is indicative of an abnormal process and in the correct clinical setting may indicate the presence of an abscess. The amount of soft tissue here should not exceed 6 mm in normality at the level of the second cervical vertebra (arrow 1). It should not exceed 14 mm at the level of the sixth cervical vertebra.

The trachea is effaced forward. This is a worrying sign as it may become compromised and narrowed (arrow 2).

Look for the epiglottis (arrow 3). In epiglottitis the epiglottis becomes enlarged and has the appearance of a thumb. This is the only abnormality seen in epiglottitis.

The amount of soft tissue in the retropharyngeal space can be increased in size in other conditions, such as cervical spine fractures.

It is also important to remember that prevertebral soft tissues can appear increased in any young child who is crying and distressed at the time of the x-ray examination, particularly if the neck is flexed – always interpret the radiographic findings taking the clinical presentation into account.

Important management points and further investigations
Immediate management

The main immediate concern is to secure the airway. If there are worrying signs such as drooling and respiratory difficulty, contact an anaesthetist immediately to intubate the child if required. An ENT surgeon should also assess the patient.

Intravenous antibiotics and fluids should be considered.

Further imaging

If the plain film is equivocal, CT of the neck with intravenous contrast is more sensitive.

Further reading

Roh J, Yoo J, Cooperman D. Cervical prevertebral soft tissue standards: a longitudinal radiographic study in a normal pediatric population. Spine J 2004;4(5, Suppl. 1):s17–8.

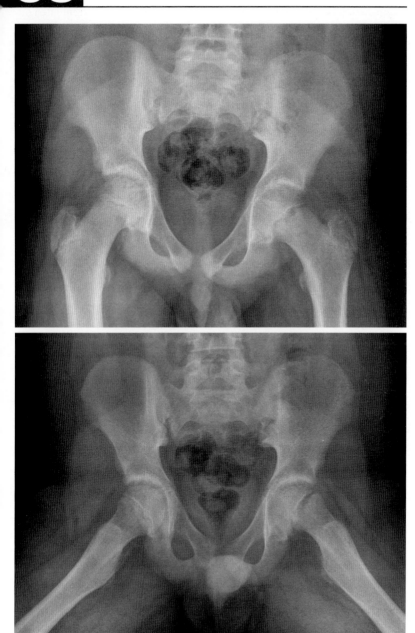

Fig. 58.1A(Top) Slipped left capital femoral epiphysis – AP view.
Fig. 58.1A(Bottom) Slipped left capital femoral epiphysis – frog-leg view.

This patient has a slip of the left capital femoral epiphysis. It is accentuated on the frog-leg view.

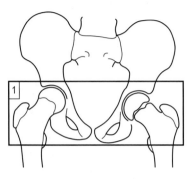 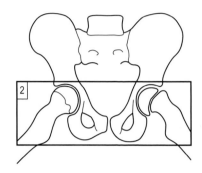

Background

The pathology is effectively a slip or fracture through the physis of the hip.

Males are affected more commonly than females in a ratio of 2.4:1, and 25% are bilateral. Obesity is a risk factor. The condition occurs in the age range 10–16 years.

The slip is posteromedial. Remember this for interpretation of the radiograph.

Clinical features

Symptoms

There may be hip, groin or knee pain. There is no history of trauma or minor trauma.

There can be a long history of limp in a chronic slip.

Signs

The patient has a limp, and may also be obese.

This condition may be encountered in A&E, general practice, orthopaedics or paediatrics.

Differential diagnosis

Remember that in the limping child the differential diagnosis is very age-dependent. This diagnosis should always be considered in the age group 10–16 years. See Chapter 59 for discussion of the limping child.

Never forget septic arthritis.

The radiographs are key to making the diagnosis.

Radiological features

Remember to assess both the AP and frog-leg lateral. The abnormalities may be accentuated on the frog-leg lateral.

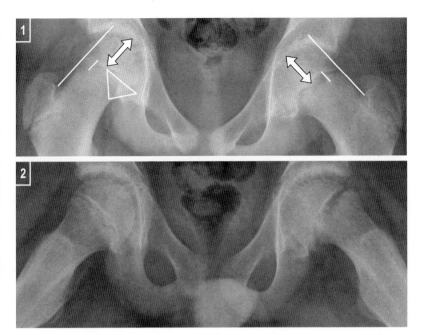

Fig. 58.1B No single sign is infallible so make all of the following assessments.

The top image is a close-up of the AP view and the bottom a close-up of the frog-leg view for comparison.

Assessment of Klein's line: This is a line drawn along the superior aspect of the femoral neck (long sloping lines). In the normal hip this line should cross the superolateral aspect of the epiphysis (see right hip), whereas in the abnormal hip it does not cross the epiphysis at all.

The epiphysis is usually narrowed on the abnormal side – this is caused by the posterior slip. In this case the epiphyseal heights are about equivalent on both sides (double-headed arrow).

The physis may also be widened (short sloping lines) and this may be accentuated on the frog-leg lateral view.

The metaphysis (femoral neck proximal to the physis) does not overlap the acetabulum on the affected side (metaphyseal exclusion sign, see triangle). On the normal side a triangle of metaphysis does overlap the acetabulum.

Important management points and further investigations

Immediate management

The patient should be referred to orthopaedics. This is not an immediate emergency.

The principles concerning septic arthritis described in the chapter on Perthes' disease (Chapter 59) apply here too.

59 | Perthes' disease

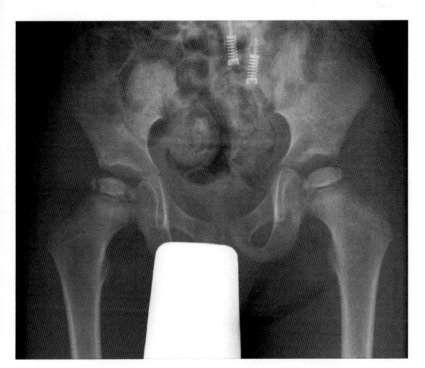

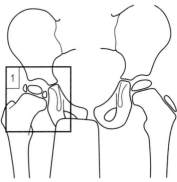

Fig. 59.1A This patient has bilateral Perthes' disease, with more marked changes on the right than the left.

Background

In Perthes' disease there is idiopathic osteonecrosis of the femoral heads. The mean age of incidence is 7 years, and boys are affected more commonly than girls in a ratio of 4:1.

It leads to osteoarthritis if not treated, and sometimes even in treated cases.

Clinical features

Symptoms

There may be hip, groin or knee pain and a limp. There is no history of trauma.

Signs

There is a decreased range of hip movements and rotation of the hip is painful. There may also be muscle spasm and atrophy.

This condition may present in A&E, paediatrics, general practice or to the orthopaedic doctor in a fracture clinic.

Differential diagnosis

- Septic arthritis is the most important (see Chapter 51).
- Slipped upper femoral epiphysis presents with hip pain but affects older children.
- Irritable hip is a self-limiting condition that affects younger children.

Remember that in the limping child the differential diagnosis is very age-dependent.

Radiological features

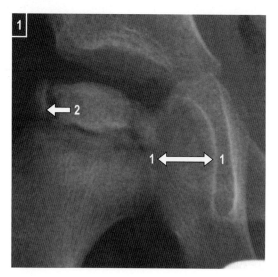

Fig. 59.1B Widening of joint space: The distance between the femoral head and the teardrop-shaped anteroinferior acetabulum is called the teardrop distance and is increased in early Perthes' disease (arrow 1).

The teardrop distance is also sensitive for the presence of a hip effusion. A discrepancy between the teardrop distances for the two hips of 1 mm or more is suggestive of an effusion.

There are subchondral lucent lines and fragmentation due to fracture (arrow 2), and also sclerosis of the epiphysis and flattening and loss of height of the epiphysis.

Important management points and further investigations
Immediate management
The limping child presents a difficult diagnostic dilemma. The likely cause is strongly influenced by the child's age, with Perthes' disease occurring between the ages of 5 and 12 years (mean 7), slipped upper femoral epiphysis in older children (teenagers) and irritable hip in toddlers.

Septic arthritis must be excluded in every limping child **as this can quickly destroy a joint.** Thus, immediate management includes blood tests to see if inflammatory markers/white cell count are raised.

Plain x-rays of the hip are indicated (see above). Ultrasound is helpful for the detection of an effusion.

Aspiration of the hip should be considered if septic arthritis is considered. This can be performed under ultrasound guidance.

A senior orthopaedic surgeon should certainly be involved in management, once your own senior has been consulted.

Further management considerations
MRI can be helpful for further diagnosis.

Follow-up should be undertaken by the orthopaedics department. These patients are at risk of secondary osteoarthritis.

Further reading
Sweeney JP, Helms CA, Minagi H, Louie KW. The widened teardrop distance: a plain film indicator of hip effusion in adults. Am J Roentgenol 1987;149:117–9.

60 Brodie's abscess

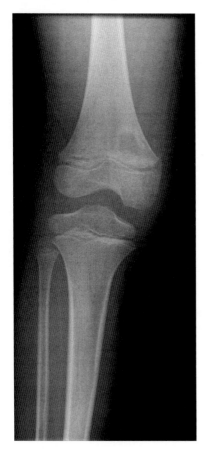

Fig. 60.1A This radiograph demonstrates a lucent lesion in the distal femoral metaphysis, with a slightly sclerotic border. This is a Brodie's abscess.

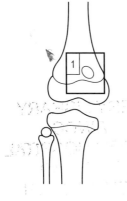

Background

Brodie's abscess is caused by subacute osteomyelitis. It occurs in children – the age range affected is wide.

Infection can spread to bone from a distant site of origin, via the haematogenous route. This is a similar mechanism to that seen in osteomyelitis.

Clinical features

Insidious in onset. There may be several months of symptoms before the diagnosis is made.

Lower limbs are more commonly affected than the upper limbs.

Symptoms

The main symptoms are pain, which may be worse at night, and a limp. Systemic symptoms such as fever are uncommon.

Signs

Localized redness and swelling occur. There may be pain on movement of the adjacent joint.

Differential diagnosis

As this condition falls somewhere between the aggressive and benign spectrum of appearances the differential diagnosis is wide, and includes tumours, eosinophilic granuloma, osteomyelitis and benign lesions such as non-ossifying fibromas.

Radiological features

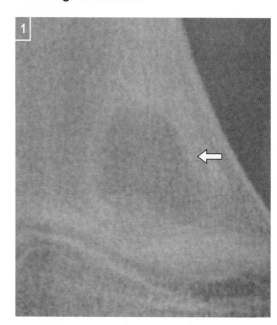

Fig. 60.1B Brodie's abscess most commonly affects the metaphysis, and the lower limb. The lesion can less commonly be epiphyseal or diaphyseal.

The lesion is lucent, well defined and may have a sclerotic border (arrow).

This is a less aggressive process than acute osteomyelitis, which is reflected in its more benign appearance (see Chapter 49 and Chapter 50).

Important management points and further investigations
Immediate management
This is an important diagnosis to make but it is not an acute emergency.

There is a considerable differential diagnosis and a paediatric radiologist may be able to help you make the diagnosis. Involve a specialist – refer to paediatric orthopaedics.

Treatment is with antibiotics, and/or surgery.

Further imaging
Several options are available, and should be instigated by a specialist:
- Bone scan is sensitive for infection, but not specific.
- CT can help differentiate from other conditions such as osteoid osteoma.
- MRI is the most sensitive modality.

61 Non-accidental injury (NAI)

NAI, or child abuse, is a topic so large and important that it merits a book in itself. Numerous complex imaging investigations may be involved. The aim of this short chapter, therefore, is not to enable the junior doctor to confidently diagnose and manage a child with suspected inflicted injury, but rather to increase the junior doctor's awareness of what unfortunately is a relatively common problem, and to help them recognize some of the appearances on plain film radiology.

If this diagnosis is suspected the radiology should be reviewed by a consultant in paediatric radiology. The condition should be managed at consultant level, with involvement of several specialties including paediatrics and radiology.

Background

Non-accidental injury should be considered with certain specific patterns of injury. A high index of suspicion is required to make the diagnosis. It is important to do so though, because if it is missed, the child may be subjected to a fatal injury the next time.

Injuries to very young children are particularly suspicious: for example, it is difficult for a non-weight-bearing child to sustain a fracture of a weight-bearing limb.

Whilst radiology is important in this condition, the diagnosis should be made on clinical and radiological grounds.

Clinical features

A thorough assessment needs to be made.

The history may be inconsistent with the injury. Does the proposed mechanism fit with what you see? Injuries include head injury (subdural haematoma), fractures (see below) and abdominal injuries.

Disabled children are at higher risk.

Differential diagnosis

Accidental injury needs to be differentiated from non-accidental injury.

Skeletal dysplasias such as osteogenesis imperfecta can also cause fractures and mimic NAI.

Radiological features

The commonest injuries seen in NAI are skeletal.

Long bone fractures are the commonest injury in NAI, but carry a low specificity. These may present to an emergency medicine junior doctor or to paediatrics, so if these patterns are suspected, senior help should be sought.

A skeletal survey will normally be performed if NAI is suspected – this consists of individual radiographs of different areas of the body.

The following injuries are suggestive of NAI:
- metaphyseal fractures – 'classic metaphyseal lesion' (CML)
- rib fractures
- skull fractures (usually encountered as part of a skeletal survey)
- fractures of differing ages (some new, some healing in the same individual).

Metaphyseal fractures (CML)

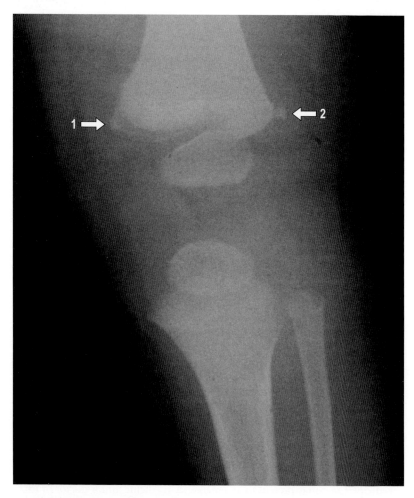

Fig. 61.1 This radiograph demonstrates two different appearances of metaphyseal fractures. These are sometimes referred to as bucket handle fractures (arrow 1) or corner fractures (arrow 2) and are highly specific for NAI. They are caused by shearing forces on the immature metaphysis. CMLs are commonest around the knee joint.

Rib fractures

Rib fractures can occur at any point along the line of the ribs, but posteromedial fractures of the rib head or neck, where the rib articulates with the vertebral body, carry high specificity for NAI as do rib fractures at different stages of healing.

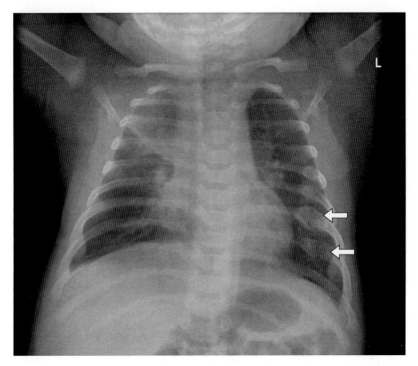

Fig. 61.2 This child has left-sided posterior rib fractures (arrows). Their orientation is often linear with respect to each other. An oblique view may help visualize lateral fractures better. This child also has consolidation in the right lung.

Rib fractures in NAI are thought to be caused by gripping and compression of the chest, with the infant held in the assailant's hands, sometimes combined with a to-and-fro shaking motion.

Skull fractures

Simple or linear skull vault fractures may be accidental or non-accidental in nature, but specificity for NAI increases the younger the patient. Complex, branching diastatic (widened) fractures and fractures that cross sutures are more specific for NAI.

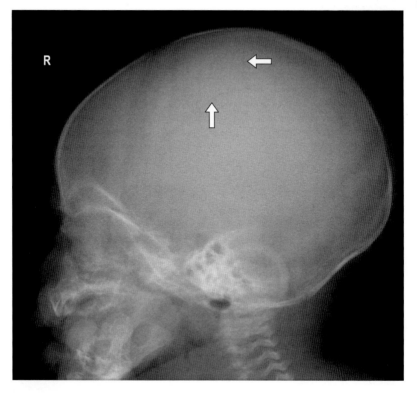

Fig. 61.3 A skull radiograph would be more likely to be performed as part of a skeletal survey. There is a skull fracture (arrows).

Important management points and further investigations

Immediate management – principles
- If you suspect non-accidental injury, inform your senior.
- Stabilize life-threatening injuries.
- Involve a senior paediatrician.
- A paediatric radiologist should be involved in helping to interpret the images.
- Referral to social services should be considered (by the team).

Further imaging

A skeletal survey may be considered to look for other injuries. A junior doctor would not normally request this.

Head injuries can be assessed in the first instance with CT or MRI. Ultrasound and/or CT can be performed to assess abdominal injuries.

Further reading

Royal College of Radiologists. Standards for radiological investigations of suspected non-accidental injury. March 2008. Available via the RCR website.

Index

Note: Page numbers followed by *f* indicate figures and *t* indicate tables.